I Chose To Live

I Chose To Live

Cancer Didn't End My Life; It Gave Me One

Scott Camacci

ISBN-13: 9780692057216
ISBN-10: 0692057218

This book is dedicated to the love of my life: my daughter Grace.

Until you came into my life, I never thought I was capable of achieving this level of fulfillment.

Your genuine warmth, intelligence, generosity, and innocence have given me immeasurable comfort and infinite inspiration.

You may never realize the impact you have had on me, each and every day.

Always be kind, always be gentle, and above all else, always be strong.

Never let anyone or anything ever hold you back from realizing your dreams.

I will always be with you.

I am you.

Contents

Chapter 1

INTRODUCTION

This is not a cancer-survivor journal. If you chose this book looking to better your prognosis with a new regimen of dried peach pits, rare Indian curry powder, and deep prayer, keep looking because you will be disappointed. I will not be going into white-blood-cell counts, C4 markers, or biopsy results. This journal is simply about ending that vacant, pit-of-your-stomach feeling that you awake to every morning, once again realizing that this was not just another bad dream. I used to have that feeling of desperation and helplessness each and every day. Then one day I woke up, and I chose not to live that way ever again. Cancer or no cancer…it was the best day of my life.

I am no different from you. I reside in the Midwest, and I have struggled all my life to become successful and earn a good salary so I can live the dream. My parents were both wonderful. They were schoolteachers who stressed education and hard work to achieve one's goals. They sent me to a small private schoolhouse out in the country during my formative years, to both give me a strong, individualized education and provide good moral guidance. Growing up in a large family in a small midwestern town, I benefitted from small-town values, but I was lucky enough to have parents who exposed me to progressive ideals. I am blessed to have five siblings and the sweetest, most beautiful daughter a father could ever hope for, named Gracie. I went to school for engineering and played the major sports. I drank with my buddies, chased girls, and loved to drive fast…but that was basically the extent of my vices.

That's my basic background…me in a nutshell. Just your average guy striving for fulfillment, pointing myself in the right direction through life, and hoping everything turns out like it should. Days turn into weeks, weeks into years, years into decades. In the winter months, you go to work in the dark and come home in the dark. So it wasn't surprising to me on that fateful day that I felt especially tired and weak, and my bones ached. *It's probably stress…no, maybe it's a lack of vitamin D…I really haven't been eating well, and I haven't seen the sun in months, so maybe that's it.*

Actually, it was none of those things. I'm not going to go into my diagnosis; suffice it to say my father died prematurely of the same condition. I really struggle these days to get vivid memories of him when he wasn't sick, when he lived life and was that strong, vibrant, inspirational man I strove to be. If only one day I could look back and deem myself lucky enough to have become a fraction of the person he had been. It's strange to me what I do remember vividly. I do remember the exact pattern of the carpet in the doctor's office when I was diagnosed…like when you remember exactly where you were when a president was shot or what you were doing when the space shuttle blew up. I was fumbling with my phone, checking e-mails, and getting more and more frustrated because I had waited for this doctor for an hour already, and I had to get out of there and get to my fantasy football draft...and right then a team of white lab coats filed into the doctor's office, and my life was never the same.

It's amazing after that day how little the daily grind now meant in the grand scheme of things. Shock, fear, and confusion were first, followed closely by months of tests and the agonizing waiting—oh my God, the waiting. Everyone has an opinion; everyone has the cure, the miracle diet, the miracle drug. You should try sniffing cinnamon or stuffing coffee grounds up your butt.

Now this was my life. The monotony of my work had been replaced with a different, much more torturous form. No longer did the guy trying to cut in front of me or the final score of last night's game mean very much.

For me, I really started to look at the big picture. Mortality will find a way to do that to you. What really became important to me were two specific things...and if you stop and think about it, they are really the only two things. How did I live my life? And how will I be remembered by my loved ones?

No matter what your condition, or if you have one at all, these two things are really all that should matter. I mentioned I was an engineer, and math has always been a big part of my life. Similarly, quantum mechanics, cosmology, and the study of the universe had always fascinated me, our origin as a species in particular. You can believe whatever you like regarding religion and creationism versus evolution, but it is irrefutable that the atoms in your body all have the same basic elements as stardust. All oxygen, carbon, and nitrogen atoms, the main ingredients that are coursing through you right now, are the same that were created in a past generation of stars over 4.5 billion years ago. To further exemplify how truly insignificant we are in our own little corner of the Milky Way: there is overwhelming evidence now, based on recent advances with NASA's Hubble and Kepler space telescopes, that there are more stars in our universe than grains of sand on every beach on Earth. The universe itself is dated to be more than thirteen billion years old, the earth over four billion. The human species, depending on your set of beliefs, is between ten thousand and two hundred thousand years old. Either way, just a speck on that time line, just a tiny blip on the radar. If I were to describe it with a golf analogy, the human species would be a one-inch gimme putt on a hole that is over a mile long.

My point here is that in relative terms, we are on this planet for a blink of an eye. How are we going to make that blink count? For me it was not going to be waiting around to see the latest glucose level. It was not going to be spent waiting around trying to get yet another CT scan. It was going to be spent getting an answer to those two most fundamental and important questions: How did I live my life? And how would I be remembered? I will not be governed by tests while I wither away into nothing. If I do, those two questions will have their answer…no, not me. No one person, nor any condition, will determine those answers but me.

Once I came to this realization on that one fateful morning…I got my life back.

So ask yourself…

How do I choose to live the remainder of my life?

How would I like to be remembered?

The vast majority of people, and such was the case with me, have never taken the time to stop and ask themselves those most fundamental questions. Our heads are buried so deep in smart phones, television, and just the rut of everyday grind, that it takes this sort of life altering slap in the face just to consider them. However, if you are truly lucky enough to one day examine those most basic realities of your time spent on earth, regardless if you have an ailment or not, than it will most certainly be time well spent.

Every person will have a unique and ultimately personalized answer to those questions. For some it may be as simple as reconciling a relationship, or accomplishing an unachieved goal. For me, I decided it was extremely important to witness and experience the destinations I had once only dreamed of seeing…and then to document those experiences so my loved ones could come along for the ride.

Now, I am not advocating ignoring your treatment, definitely to the contrary. I don't have a death wish; I have a wish to live life. For me it was very important to do everything I could do to preserve my quality of life for as long as possible. That meant coming up with a strategy to plan my adventures, spacing my travels out, and timing them in such a manner that I could schedule the best possible health care, along with the ultimate goal of being at my absolute strongest as I departed for my next adventure. It might seem tough to manage…it was not.

And so I began my life.

Chapter 2

2.1 MARANELLO

taly is a feast for the senses. Is it any wonder that this destination would be one of my primary goals? Artistic inspiration and daring innovation accompany every breadth of this spectacular country. The Renaissance challenged world views based on contributions from names that have spanned the generations: Donatello, Da Vinci, architecture by Brunelleschi, and the magnificent masterpieces of Michelangelo, just to name the obvious. The cultural, scientific, and intellectual reformation had begun in Italy, and the world was never the same as a result. That is why I had to start here, where the embodiment of what I was feeling was pursued as a lifestyle every day. Italy still does—now in a more capitalistic way, of course—embody these same daring and artistic axioms hailing from the golden age of rebirth. From the clothes they wear to the food they eat, every aspect of their lives is an artistic and daring expression of their flair and their desire to live and experience life to the fullest...right down to the works of art they fashion out of steel and carbon fiber. I am of course talking about the legendary coach builder and Formula 1 race-car team, Ferrari. And this is where my first adventure begins.

So I boarded a nonstop flight to Bologna. You will notice that I seem to be going to some very expensive and exotic locations, and they may seem spontaneous in nature. Not the case...I planned out everything I wanted to do and how I was going to afford to do it. Even before my diagnosis, I had already decided early on I wanted to leave whatever I could of value to my daughter. So I streamlined everything I owned into my major investment, basically stock and property (my home). Everything else I decided was just frivolous, so I sold all my crap. I really didn't need, or even use, half of the toys or junk memorabilia I had collected over the years. I have seen from experience, if those things are lying around after you've dearly departed, they will just cause fights among loved ones trying to either divide or liquidate them. Now, is that the memory you want to leave behind? So I sold all my junk, cashed in a few airline miles, liquidated a couple of IRAs, and now I'm at thirty thousand feet.

It's weird…I used to be afraid of heights and uneasy when flying. It doesn't seem to be that big a deal anymore in the grand scheme of things. If you decide to depart on these adventures, you will notice that to become a common occurrence. The little things, the annoying glitches to your day, just don't matter anymore. You will get in an elevator, and instead of there being a weird, uncomfortable silence for thirty seconds while you wonder what this person's story is, you might now just blurt out hello. Because what does it really matter, right? Who knows where it might go? Directions, a common friend, who knows? We're here for a blink of an eye, remember?

You will also notice that the chapters I decided to include in this book, or journal, or whatever you want to call this, are fairly hair-raising and adrenaline charged in nature. I went on several trips that were not, but they were not nearly as fun to recall or write as these. So here goes…

We took a hard bank left, and into view came the never-ending rows of terra-cotta roofs in the city center tapering away into the perfectly geometrical shapes of the Italian farmers' fields. Winding their way through these fields and into the mountainous terrain were the most exquisite serpentine roads you have ever laid eyes on, and they were the very reason I had chosen Bologna.

I had no plans on just taking the ho-hum Autostrada from Bologna to Modena, where my target, the Aerautodromo Modena Spa, resides (Ferrari factory racetrack). There is a specific set of roads through the hills backing up to Bologna that make up some of the most challenging anywhere in the world. Hairpin turns and blistering corners, followed by a tight series of chicanes and then near-perfect straightaways where you can let loose the beast of an engine that resides within.

As I stated earlier, I did my homework before I planned these excursions, and this first trip was definitely not the exception. My love for cars, especially exotic and European cars, came at the very young age of twelve while attempting to rebuild a Fiat Spider in our backyard. The car I decided on renting in Bologna and driving to Modena was definitely no throwback to my childhood four-cylinder anemic excuse for a convertible. It was in fact Maranello's newest and most exhilarating of their models, the flagship Ferrari Spider. This spaceship of a Ferrari boasts a dual-clutch twin turbo V-8 that goes north of 660 hp at 8,000 rpm and does 0 to 60 in three seconds flat with a top speed of 205 miles per hour (330 kilometers per hour). Basically, for the layperson, it goes faster on four wheels than most competitive motorcycles can do on two. However, this rocket is far from exclusively offering speed and neck-breaking acceleration. The primary allure of Ferrari throughout the generations has typically been its body design. The Pinninfarina design studio gave birth to the flowing, aerodynamic curves that accentuate their low, wide stance and give every one of these prancing horses their unique form and immediate recognition. This beauty is no exception, with its short, muscular front end swooping artistically through its midriff and eventually dumping into a huge engine-cooling vent that you need to keep small children and animals away from in fear that they might be sucked in. The rear quarter then wraps around its extremely bulbous rear end, in such a manner that the famous artist Rubens, himself known in Renaissance Italy for capturing similarly beautiful curves, could only be jealous of.

The only time I've felt safer than sliding into that beautifully hand-stitched, leather-wrapped, carbon-fiber seat that absolutely envelops your entire upper torso, was coming home after the first long, rainy day of middle school and having my mother wrap her arms around me and promise everything would be OK. But this was no longer middle school. When I pushed the button for engine start, I appeared to be in the cockpit of an F-16 fighter jet. Attempting to ignore a red "LAUNCH" button next to my right thigh that I thought might eject me, I lightly nudged the accelerator, and the 660 hp twin turbo engine roared to life behind me. There would be no Led Zeppelin or Jay-Z on this trip…I didn't even care where the radio was. With the turbos singing in tenor and the dual exhaust switching between baritone and bass, the most beautiful music I had ever heard was only a light touch of the pedal away.

So I sped off toward the hills of Bologna on my way to Modena. It was on its way to twilight and then to dusk as I headed toward the winding hills backing up to Bologna. I was taking the Ferrari through its paces, negotiating turns, braking hard into corners, trying to get a good feel for the car and where she would break loose, before I got to the most demanding portion of the road. As the sun tickled the nearby mountaintops, my heart started pounding as I accelerated toward the first hairpin turn. Negotiating a line that I felt would give me the best acceleration on the exit, I dived into the corner and stomped on the brakes, feeling the ABS hydraulics pulsating beneath my foot and the massive Brembo ceramic rotors bringing all thirty-four hundred pounds of sheer testosterone to a near-dead halt. Now I switched back to the accelerator and noticed as I powered out of the corner that there were multiple patches of rubber leading directly into the ditch, showing others' fates who did not fare as well as me. As I peered ahead, I could not have been more delighted to see the road straighten almost to the horizon. I pinned the accelerator to the floor, and my head was violently thrown back as the turbos whistled and the exhaust spat fire and inhaled a huge breath, crackling and roaring at the same time. I shifted the paddle to third, then fourth, and then fifth, the LED lights on the steering wheel beaming impatiently at me to shift at each red line. The countryside became a blur, like an acrylic landscape painting full of muddled earth tones. As I looked down, I saw I was at 230 kilometers per hour as I hit sixth gear. The dashed center line on the street had now been transformed by speed into solid, as I approached the top of a slight and steady rise in the road.

As I eclipsed the rise, I hit seventh gear and at the same time saw a pair of tiny headlights approaching very rapidly, which is what tends to happen at 160 miles per hour. As I approached the headlights, to my dismay, another set of lights appeared, only these were alternating blue and red lights accompanied by the all-too-familiar screeching European siren. Every muscle in my body tensed up as I passed the Italian police car as quickly as it had appeared, and now he had disappeared over the same crest of the hilltop I had just eclipsed.

I don't know what came over me; I have no idea if it was the adrenaline or the fact that I had no idea what would happen to me getting caught doing 100 miles per hour over the speed limit. I don't know what it was…but I didn't hit the brake; I hit the gas.

It felt like an hour had gone by, but realistically it was probably about twenty seconds before in my rear view, I saw the blue lights turn around and come back over the hilltop. I even convinced myself they would never try to catch up to me at the pace I was moving…wrong. I was now going almost 185 miles per hour and approaching civilization again fast. I definitely did not want to put anyone else's safety at risk, so I had to do something, and quick. As I approached town and had to slow up, I saw the blue lights quickly closing the gap. I abruptly made a right turn off the main road as soon as their lights disappeared behind another rise in the road so they wouldn't be able to see my brake lights. I approached what looked to be a small village of maybe a few hundred people. I coasted into town so as not to raise any suspicion with my loud exhaust. I killed my lights and crept onto a street with about five homes all lined up, one after the next. All the houses had street-level garages, and I noticed one of them had its garage doors open. My heart was ready to come out of my chest at this point, and I didn't know if it was my blood pressure or the exhaust that was causing the ringing in my ears, but remarkably, I still had my wits about me. I snuck the car into the open garage, hopped out, and shut the doors behind me as quietly as I could. I tiptoed out of the garage and huddled next to the door, peering frantically at the main road to see where the police car was. Had they seen me get off the main road? Did they see my brake lights?

I couldn't even breathe as I saw the police car approach the intersection, not even a football field away from where I had turned off. To my utter amazement, the police car kept going on the main road, not even slowing down for the intersection. After about three or four minutes, the blue lights had completely vanished. I knelt down to catch my breath and get my shit together for a few minutes.

Once I had regained what little composure I had left, I opened the doors and pushed the car out of the garage, not wanting the Ferrari's exhaust to awaken the homeowner's suspicion like some startled, barking dog. I waited about thirty minutes. I didn't see one other vehicle the whole time, so I decided to backtrack and take the Autostrada to Modena.

Do not get me wrong. I'm not condoning for a minute running from police in a foreign country. I should still be rotting in an Italian jail cell. What I am saying is that you need to fulfill the dreams you have always had and take the risks that lead to their fulfillment. Now, was it watching the movie *The Cannonball Run* literally fifty times in a row and marveling at the Lamborghini accelerating away from the early '80s police car that made me hit the gas? I'm not sure…but it's a fantasy I have always had. Let's just from this point forward keep the authorities out of the equation. You can't make many dreams come true waiting for Amnesty International to get you out of a reckless driving arrest.

Needless to say, the next day at the Ferrari racetrack was far more anticlimactic. Yes, it was fun. I spent a half day putting the Ferrari through its paces, but after the previous night's excitement, I was ready to get to Florence and partake in the more cultural and artistic elements of my Italian excursion.

2.2 MEDICI

I opened the convertible roof and decided on a more scenic route through the rolling hills of the Modena province, passing through quaint little villages and towns such as Pievepelago and Abetone. Enjoying every minute of the winding roads and the open-aired motoring experience, I stopped a couple of times for cappuccino and once at a roadside gelato stand.

As I descended into Florence from the hills on the serpent-like Tuscany roads, the homes started getting closer and closer together and more majestic in architecture...three and four stories with terraces and terracotta clay tiles. As I entered the city center via the more and more frequent roundabouts, I made my way through the narrowing streets to the historic district on the way to my hotel.

As I exited another small alley-sized road between two small cafés, I was awestricken by the size and majesty of the Palazzo Vecchio. With its massive thirteenth-century castle-like archi-tecture, this museum still serves as Florence's town hall and overlooks one of Michelangelo's statues of David. Both Da Vinci and Michelangelo were commissioned to adorn the inner walls of the Palazzo Vecchio with their original frescos.

After a nearly four-hour drive, I had finally negotiated the many confusing piazzas and street signs and made it through the historical district (which I would later find I needed a permit for) to my hotel. My pace now much more resembled that of the walking dead than of an anxious tourist.

I stumbled into the main entrance and was stopped in my tracks. Before me was the most breathtaking entrance to a building I had ever witnessed. The entire lobby was fashioned from marble, with massive ornate chandeliers that looked like they had been placed there four or five centuries ago and would last for four or five more. I walked down a series of winding staircases to the main floor, while marveling at the giant works of Rubenesque art adorning every square inch of wall space. I made my way over to a person who resembled someone who might be working there to ask if I had somehow made a wrong turn into one of Florence's abundant art galleries. With a chuckle and a familiar nod, as if he had been asked the same question a dozen times that night, he pointed me toward what looked to be the front desk of the hotel.

The suites were also very impressive, as you would see if you walked into a master bedroom in a Tuscan villa. Decorative armoires from the previous century made of dark walnut with maple inlays were the first thing that caught the eye, followed by tapestries on the walls, an ornate iron-sculpted pedestal bed, and finally the cherubs holding up both heavy glass tables, and dimly lit sconces on the walls. I passed out the minute my head hit the pillow…thanking my lucky stars that I was on Egyptian cotton sheets and a feather bed, not on a concrete floor in a jail cell.

My first morning in Florence was spectacular. Freshly cut roses and white lilies were both a part of the first breath I took as I exited my suite on the way to the hotel's rooftop terrace. I climbed a long and narrow winding spiral staircase up the fifteenth-century turret that eventually opened into a flower- and ivy-laden pergola. Ducking down to avoid the foliage, I entered the gateway to the portico, which opened up into one of the most magnificent and inspiring views I had ever been lucky enough to witness. In every direction, as far as the eye could see, there was one iconic Italian landmark after the next. In the distance, and marking the traveler's northernmost point of Florence's historic district, was the majestic and column-laden fourteenth-century Piazza Della Liberta. I spun to my left and was met by Brunelleschi's Basilica di Santo Spirito, filled with masterpieces and a golden baroque alter. To the east sat the famous galleries that have remained a domicile for centuries to Michelangelo's *David* and sculptures by Da Vinci and Donatello. But they all pale in comparison to what I was squinting on this bright sunny morning to get a glimpse of. A chill went up my spine as I laid eyes on what I had been searching the horizon for. Across the banks of the Arno river, the river that knifes its way through the downtown corridor, lies the home of the most historic collection of Renaissance masterpieces ever assembled, the extraordinary Uffizi Gallery.

The Uffizi (or "offices" in English) was built as headquarters for the Florentine magistrates of the Renaissance period, specifically the Medici ruling family who not only owned the largest bank in Europe, but whose famous ancestor *Medico di Potrone* is also believed to be the first "medical" doctor (Medici being plural for Medico). The Medici family's dynasty rose to be widely regarded as the most prestigious patron to the arts in recorded history...and the Uffizi Gallery represents and houses all the work that the Medici Empire ever commissioned.

As I stood mesmerized by the view, taking in the history and imagining what it might have been like to live in the era of the golden rebirth, I felt a tug on my shoulder. It was Vincenzo, the same hotel employee I had spoken to the previous night. I quickly realized I had that same vacant look on my face that he had witnessed last night when I thought I had mistakenly stumbled into a Florentine art gallery. In his broken English and with a sarcastic slap on the back, he uttered, "I see you look sleepy again."

We both had a good laugh, and then I was off to the Uffizi. I decided to cross the Arno River on foot over yet another example of history that the Medici family can be credited for. The Ponte Santa Trinita (or Holy Trinity) claims the privileged designation as the oldest elliptical arched bridge in existence today. Cosimo Medici, the most powerful duke of the 1560s, commissioned the most highly respected architect of his day, Bartolomeo

Ammannati, to build Michelangelo's vision of artistic structure and strength. The peaks of each arch were adorned with the Medici zodiac, and in 1608 sculptures were also added to each of the points of the bridge's entry with the artist's interpretation of the seasons…spring, summer, autumn, and winter.

I made my way to the entrance of the Uffizi Gallery, and the line for general admission wrapped around the U-shaped museum. I am not going to spend much time describing this gallery or the masterpieces stored within. This experience is something that words cannot aptly describe, and if there is any takeaway from this book at all, it is to visit personally these wonders the world has to offer and not read about them in books like this one or Google the statue of David. I think what I am trying to describe here is most succinctly and eloquently explained in the movie *Good Will Hunting*, where Robin Williams explains to the academic genius Matt Damon that "if the subject of art is brought up, you could probably recite the theory of every art book that has ever been written. If Michelangelo is discussed…you could probably describe his life's work, political aspirations, and relationship to the pope, the whole works. But I bet you can't tell me what it smells like in the Sistine Chapel. You've never actually looked up and stared at that beautiful ceiling."

So that is my only point. I can't explain this gallery to you or even how the humidity feels in a tropical rain forest...you just have to go out there and experience it for yourself. And don't wait; do it now.

I will, however, touch on one painting because it was so inspirational. It is Parmigianino's *Madonna with the Long Neck*. Standing nearly eight feet tall, Ferdinando de' Medici, grand prince of Tuscany, purchased it in 1698, and it now stands in the Uffizi. This particular painting is known for the artist's impression of the Madonna having an elongated neck and fingers, almost queen-like features. It was known then and now as "mannerism" style, and it challenged the high Renaissance style of perfect symbiotic composition, which was the popular style of the day. It led to artists such as Parmigianino being known as trendsetters and actually being referred to as the first "modernist" painters...which is exactly why I decided to bring up this painting, and this painting alone.

Parmigianino and artists like him in that era ignited a culture in Italy of trendsetting and boldness that is still inherent in Italy's fashion, gastronomy, art, and engineering to this very day. And now you and I are the beneficiaries…

2.3 MADONNA

I made my way back to the hotel after the Uffizi with the intent of trying out the hotel restaurant for my final dinner. I showered and decided to change into a suit, because I was told it was a rather fancy establishment. I was not misinformed and was actually pleasantly surprised at the decor being more modern and cozy at the same time, almost like a library. I had read the reviews online and was convinced I needed to try the Mediterranean Sea bass and mushroom risotto. Actually, Mediterranean Sea bass with Venus rice, oysters, and herbs grown locally in Tuscany was the entrée of choice. When you experience truly authentic Italian cuisine, there is no parallel to the senses. The only thing that could make the experience any better was the right pairing of wine. In an attempt to keep the wine local to Florence, I decided to try the wine Tuscany is most widely renowned for: Chianti. There are over 150,000 acres dedicated to the Chianti grape in Tuscany. An aged Chianti Riserva is best, because it has to be stored for more than three years to receive that designation. I had read earlier that 2001 was supposed to be one of the best years for the Sangiovese grape, which must make up at least 75 percent of the Chianti grape blend. I was thrilled to notice on the menu a 2001 Da Vinci Chianti Riserva, which seemed very appropriate to round out my once-in-a-lifetime experience at the Uffizi Gallery.

As I sliced into the first sea bass filet, I surveyed the room and briefly glanced up toward the bar area. I suddenly dropped my knife and fork so loudly on my plate that other patrons turned around to see what sort of collision had just happened. Standing at the bar was the most stunning, statuesque vision of a woman I think I had ever seen. I'd had only two sips of wine to that point, so I know I wasn't buzzed and seeing things…so just to make sure, I blinked a couple of times in case my contacts had fogged over. It was now apparent she was real. She was in a tight red form-fitting dress with long brown hair to the middle of her back, with eyes so strikingly blue they were noticeable at my distance of thirty yards. She literally could have just walked off a *Vogue* cover shoot, towering over her girl-friend, so she was at least five feet ten in bare feet. And now she was looking in my direction, I was sure in order to see what klutz had caused all this commotion. When our eyes met, I literally gasped at their brilliance and must have looked like a deer in headlights.

The spell was quickly broken as I noticed this same guy from the hotel, Vincenzo, walk up to the girls from behind the bar and ask them what they would like to drink. He muttered something in Italian to them while they all looked in my direction and giggled. Does this hotel have, like, only one employee? I tried to gather myself and swallow the last bit of fish so I wouldn't choke, which I'm sure would have guaranteed an even more entertaining evening for everyone at this point. I must have looked like a second grader after being told to finish his last chicken strip before he could watch his favorite cartoon. I hurriedly wiped my face with my napkin while I searched my lapel for a piece of gum. I took a couple of deep breaths to calm myself a bit and to talk myself into going up to the bar. Before this trip and prior to this new state of mind, I would have never taken the risk. Not anymore...

I told my waiter I would be right back, tossed the napkin aside, and started up toward the bar. To my dismay, my new soulmate and her girlfriend were now both nowhere to be seen. I started muttering obscenities under my breath on the way up to the bar now. The people I passed, who had seen my earlier clumsiness, must have thought I had some form of Tourette's. I finally made it to the bar, and Vincenzo was pouring a drink for another couple on the opposite end of the restaurant. As soon as he finished, and we made eye contact, he started over toward me with a shit-eating grin on his face. When he got about halfway to me, I said, at a volume reserved for misbehaving kids at the park, "Vince! What did you say to them about me?", recalling my earlier escapades with the cutlery. I was scowling at him now, but he seemed to be looking right through me. Then from behind me I heard a soft but heavy Italian accent reply, "He said you always have that look on your face." I froze and squeezed my eyes shut in embarrassment. My shoulders shrugged up instinctively as I slowly turned around to see that she was right behind me during my outburst to Vincenzo…she and her girlfriend must have just come back from the bathroom. I readied myself for the abuse I was about to take and slowly opened my eyes. She and her friend grabbed each other and just about fell over laughing.

All I could do was stand there and shake my head, waiting for them to resuscitate. Eventually they caught their breath and stood back up visibly shaken from all the laughter at my expense. I was right about her being five feet ten, because I'm six feet two, and with the four-inch heels, she was now looking straight at me, a foot away, with those mesmerizing blue eyes. Vincenzo must have realized I was about to stutter out some dumb comment, so fortunately he took the reins and introduced me. Her name was Madonna. I immediately was struck by how coincidental it was that I had just been captivated earlier that same day by Parmigianino's painting possessing the same name. So, of course, I tried explaining that to Madonna, and she in turn translated that to her friend, Maria. Now, I don't speak much Italian, but I have become pretty proficient at ordering food in Italian, so I immediately recognized the word *"formaggio"* in Maria's response right before they again started into a fit of laughter. Madonna must have noticed that I had caught the Italian word for "cheesy" in Maria's reply by the look on my face, because all of a sudden I could tell that she felt bad about her laughter, and she asked if she could buy me a drink. I politely declined, let them know that it was a pleasure meeting them, and went back to my table to finish my dinner.

Now, I get the feeling that not too many people turn down drinks offered to them by Madonna in the red dress…because now she was on somewhat of a mission. As I was settling up my check at my table, the waiter came over with a large piece of tiramisu with two forks, and following closely behind was Madonna. She asked if she could join me, and of course I accepted but asked where Maria had gone. She explained that she had to wake up early, so she had to leave, but Maria wanted me to know she was sorry about her comment and didn't mean anything by it. I told her it was nothing and that it took a whole lot more than that to get me flustered these days.

As the tiramisu slowly disappeared, I learned that Madonna worked in the fashion industry during the day but also was a hostess at this same hotel restaurant in the evenings and on weekends to supplement her income, as well as getting a break on her apartment next door that the hotel owned. We ordered a couple more glasses of Chianti as we discussed her background and my visit to her beautiful country. Hours must have passed, because the next time I forced myself to break away from her gaze, I realized we were the last table occupied, and most of the employees had left. I walked her out of the restaurant, through the museum disguised as a hotel lobby, and out onto the cobblestone path toward her flat. We arrived at her door as I explained that my flight left at noon the next day and how much I had enjoyed my last night there in her company. She gave me a light kiss on the cheek, and we said good night.

I was awoken later that night by a light knocking on the door of my suite.

I missed my noon flight but caught the next at four o'clock.

Chapter 3

If ever there were a setting that filled your imagination with the exotic, from the black sandy beaches to the tales of virgins being thrown into the volcanoes to appease the gods, Hawaii would be that place. Madame Pele, more widely referred to as the "Fire Goddess," is the fabled goddess of fire, lightning, and wind. According to Polynesian mythology, she was the creator of the Hawaiian Islands. So how could this romanticized archipelago of eight individual islands not be on my list? More specifically, how could the big island of Hawaii not be, where the Fire Goddess lives and breathes to this very day?

I am speaking of course of Kilauea. The most active of the volcanoes in the Hawaiian Island chain, Madame Pele gave birth to her second youngest a mere one hundred thousand years ago. Kilauea was thought for generations to be a satellite to its much larger neighbor Mauna Loa, but recent geographical surveys and eruptive history not coinciding proved otherwise. Kilauea's summit sits at four thousand feet above sea level, and due to its highly publicized recent activity, it easily made it to the top of my list when I was planning out my travel itinerary.

I flew into Honolulu International, as most tourists do, admiring the views of the enormous extinct crater within Diamondhead on our approach. I subsequently boarded an island-hopper prop plane to fly to Hilo on the big island of Hawaii, the recent mecca of volcanists in the United States. The reason for my heightened excitement to get to Kilauea first, not to mention all the local publicity, was surrounding a very recent development in its topographical landscape. Where the volcano's surface flow of lava finally leaks into the ocean, a huge portion of the cliff had collapsed onto itself, and now a veritable fire hose of lava was spraying into the Pacific. I had only heard stories of what the visual might be like to witness this in person, so I was eager to get to my hotel and get some sleep so that I was fresh for what promised to be a strenuous hike the next day.

I slept late into the afternoon the next day, I could only assume mostly due to jet lag. That was OK, though, as my plans for the day were to just have a hearty lunch and then drive to a hiking trail near the former town of Kalapana on the southeast side of the island. From this vantage point, it would only be about a five-mile hike to the ocean entry. I quickly ate lunch and then jumped in my rental to drive to Kalapana. When I finally arrived, I parked in a lot near the trailhead and got geared up for my nearly ten-mile round-trip hike. There's something I need to explain, because now it was close to five o'clock, and the sun set around 7:40 p.m., and it takes way longer than two and a half hours to hike ten miles over a bed of lava.

Again, I researched this hike quite a bit, and I concluded that the absolute best experience was to be had at night. It might sound a bit crazy or naïve to hike unfamiliar lava beds at night, but I came prepared with a light worn on your head and a flashlight, along with GPS, of course, so I felt pretty safe…plus, Madame Pele would have no interest in me.

So I packed up and started out toward the lava flow. The first mile or so is really just a dirt road before you start to come to the lava beds laid down decades earlier. Really the only way to describe the beds from a distance would be if you have ever seen a forest right after a California wildfire. It has a desolate, almost moonscape-like quality, with the exception of the lava bed itself. There are very distinct patterns of flow, almost if a river had stopped flowing and solidified into charcoal. As the lava hardens, huge crevices open up, some a few inches, some a few feet, so I could already tell I was in for a long and potentially dangerous hike back in the dark. As you start to walk on the lava, you can definitely feel a difference in texture the farther inland you go. I was told later that this was due to the age of the lava; the newer it was, the crispier it sounded beneath my boots. Earlier I used the term "former town" of Kalapana for good reason. In the late '80s and early '90s, flows from the Kupaianaha vent of Kilauea crept into this town and first burned it to the ground and then buried it. A nearby subdivision was also decimated and now lies under fifty feet of hardened lava. This portion of the hike was definitely not the highlight, as you could almost feel the heartache of the townspeople whose homes once stood right beneath your feet.

Every step from here on needed to be careful and calculated…I wasn't sure when this lava bed was going to transition from hard to molten. There was smoke nearby now, gas to be more accurate, sulfur dioxide specifically, that was being released from the molten magma. This gas is toxic and can irritate a healthy person's lungs, and it even can do real damage to someone suffering from an existing breathing ailment. As I ventured farther toward the ocean, at approximately three miles in, I came upon my first molten surface flow.

It was glowing red like a piece of intensely heated charcoal. As I got within ten yards, I started to feel the intense heat as you would when you approach a large bonfire. There was a large ridge of oozing magma glowing intensely at the front of the flow, cooling quickly to black lava rock as it progressed. The best way I could describe it is when I was a kid during the Fourth of July, lighting the little pellets of charcoal snakes. They would grow long black tails as the embers near the source glowed red, feeding the snake until it was two feet long. This sort of resembled the flow I now witnessed. I couldn't bear to get within a couple of feet because of the intense heat, as well as not wanting to get splashed with magma so intensely heated that it liquefies rock.

I could see now that evening was approaching quickly, so I carefully followed the molten ridge to where it had crept the furthest. I rounded its farthermost point and was then on my way to my ultimate destination of the Pacific cliffs at Komukuna, where Kilauea was pouring its fiery display into the ocean. All the while I had to be extremely cognizant of where there were small outcroppings of liquid magma. Now almost all the crevices that receded into hardened lava were filled with seething red liquid rock.

I was now within a couple of football fields of the Pacific, and I could see in the distance a huge plume of white steam emanating from below the cliffs. As I approached I could now see a glow of light from behind the cliffs, almost like a sunrise before it breaches the horizon.

I wasn't really prepared for what I saw next. It was as if Niagara Falls were filled full of molten lava, but now its velocity was increased three-fold, gushing into the ocean below, exploding and popping like popcorn when it hit the Pacific's surface. The only thing I could remotely liken it to would be watching workers in a steel foundry pour a steaming cauldron of liquid metal into a mold…only this was on a much more titanic scale. I just sat down right there on the edge of the cliff as the sun set, mesmerized by earth's incredible display of formation and rebirth.

I lost track of time, but I think about an hour had passed of my being spellbound by what I was witnessing. I decided it would likely be a good idea to start heading back so that I didn't lose my focus due to fatigue. I switched on my head-light and started the long trek back to Kalapana. I must have hiked about a half mile back when I turned around to see how far I was from the cliffs. I turned off my light to get a better look.

I couldn't believe my eyes. I had to sit down again to revel in what only could be described as a near-religious experience. The stars were the most brilliantly lit I had ever observed, and com-bined with that was this sea of glowing lava, filled by rivers of luminous magma. I imagined that this was as close as I would ever get to being present for the birth of our planet, when in its infancy, Earth was a seething fireball of volcanic and earth-shaping tectonics, while being showered with mountain-sized meteors and comets. I sat there for about another hour and then reluctantly headed back, basically now floating from the spectacle that Mother Nature had just afforded me.

The next morning I awoke in my hotel in Hilo, once again excited for what the day had in store. Today I was going to the summit of Mauna Kea, its peak being the highest point on all the Hawaiian Islands. A dormant volcano now, it stands close to fourteen thousand feet above sea level, and if measured from its oceanic base, it is taller than Mount Everest. However, the view is not the primary reason for my interest in Mauna Kea; it's actually what was built on top of it, the Keck Observatory.

My drive to the summit proved to be interesting in and of itself. From Hilo to the summit, you traverse just about every ecosystem that exists on the Big Island. Starting with the tropical-rainforest-like climate of Hilo, you quickly pass through the native trees of 'Ohi'a Lehua. These cactus-like trees with their beautiful red blossoms are indigenous and unique to the Big Island, while representing Hawaii as their official tree. As you pass the halfway point, and your odometer clicks to about twenty miles from Hilo, you start your ascent. First you pass a plethora of cattle ranches on the way, marked with signs to avoid the "invisible cows." Apparently on cloudy days, these open-range farms can prove dangerous, as their livestock can suddenly appear in front of your vehicle through the mist of a low-lying cloud.

As you continue about the windy road, the ranches become fewer and farther between, and you can actually feel the air start to thin. The view starts to get more and more inviting as you steadily climb past sixty-five hundred feet. At ninety-two hundred feet you are encouraged to stop at the Onizuka Center for International Astronomy, renamed after the Hawaii-born astronaut Ellison Onizuka, who died in the *Challenger* disaster. This brief respite is not only to take a look at the incredible views but more importantly to acclimatize your body before the final climb to the summit. A minimum of thirty minutes is recommended to wait at this elevation to avoid altitude sickness (puking your guts out) at the top. It's a good thing I didn't scuba dive the day before, because summiting would have been out of the question.

After my thirty-minute acclimation, I jumped back in the car and was ready for the final ascent. I was correctly advised to rent an all-wheel drive vehicle, because now the road turned to gravel and increased in grade. As I neared the summit, there was a drastic change in temperature, now registering on the car's thermostat at below freezing. This must have been accurate, because as I rounded a turn, the summit came into view, with its multiple peaks covered in snow…Snow in Hawaii?!

As I approached the observatories, I passed a massive radio telescope with a dish that must have exceeded eighty feet in diameter. As I reached the summit, I now had an amazing 360-degree view, including a fantastic view of Waimea and even the Island of Maui. The road signs now warned to slow to five miles per hour so as to prevent your vehicle from stirring up dust. The landscape up here once again, was much like you would expect to see on the moon. I drove a few hundred more yards past the twin Subaru observatories, and then into view came my ultimate destination, the Keck Observatory.

If you are at all interested in astronomy or cosmology like I am, then Keck is the Holy Grail. Standing eight stories tall, each of the two Keck telescopes weigh close to three hundred tons each. The twin thirty-three-foot mirrored telescopes are the largest in the world, and even more impressive than that are the active optics systems that are employed. Each mirror consists of thirty-six individual segments that adjust up to two thousand times per second to an accuracy of 1/25,000 the thickness of a human hair. The Keck beams a guided laser into the sky, allowing these adaptive optics to adjust to the aberrations of the earth's atmosphere. What this translates to is the clearest and most powerful telescope on the planet today. Keck is responsible for discovering planets in other solar systems that orbit stars similar to our own. This allows us to pinpoint which planet might have conditions similar to our own in order to support life. Keck also has been able to confirm what had long been theorized, that our Milky Way galaxy orbits around a supermassive black hole that is twenty-six thousand light-years away, which translates to approximately 24.7 quintillion miles.

With my nerdy appetite now satisfied, I hiked over to one of the many peaks on top of the summit, my breath now visible from the below-freezing temperature. I looked down, and now a sea of clouds had formed thousands of feet below. You feel as if you are on top of the world as you look down into the ocean of clouds churning and waving beneath your feet. I felt like this was as close to being in space as one could get without being an astronaut.

As the sun set quickly beneath my feet, I gazed around in wonder as the stars appeared, so vibrant and close now that it made me reflect on the night before. This is what was so unique and awe-inspiring about the Hawaiian Islands… on virtually the same day, you could be witnessing molten earth spewing from the core of our planet and then literally only be a couple of hours' drive from the pinnacle of the earth, feeling like you could reach out and touch the heavens. Once again I sat there by myself in amazement and self-reflection, gazing at the stars.

3.2 KAUAI

The next morning I was bound for the garden isle of Kauai. I once again boarded a prop plane island hopper, and within an hour I was landing in Lihue. Everything is only an hour away on the Hawaiian Islands, either by car or by plane. Once I picked up my rental car, I was an hour's drive away from the resort I would be staying at in Princeville, on Kauai's northeast shore. As I drove down the island's east coast, I thought to myself that at some point you can get almost numb or, dare I say, "used to" the beauty of these islands, but Kauai is a step above. The lush and majestic landscape that encompasses this island once again is beyond my ability to put into words and must be experienced in person to truly appreciate. Formed by the volcanic explosion of Mount Wai'ale'ale five million years ago, this now-dormant mountain terrain epitomizes the term "rain forest." At its summit, Mount Wai'ale'ale holds the record for the wettest place on earth, averaging almost five hundred inches of annual rainfall.

On my way to the hotel, my only stop was at a small snorkel rental store just outside Princeville.

Not only was the landscape magnificent on Kauai's north shore, but the coral reefs were supposed to be equally impressive, and I intended to see that for myself.

One more blissful night's sleep in paradise and I was on my way to Ke'e Beach on the north shore. This is the last beach before the Nā Pali Coast and the only beachline that remains traversable by foot; from that point on, it is sheer volcanic cliffs covered in an abundance of lush vegetation. This beach was near the trailhead of my hike planned for the following day, so I wanted to scout it out. Ke'e is also renowned for snorkeling in its coral reefs. As you pull into the lot at Ke'e Beach, you are immediately struck by how untouched by humans the environment still seems to be. A dense line of palm trees edges the beach as large waves crash above the coral.

As I walked along the beach in the midday sun, now in the mid-eighties, I came upon a relatively flat outcropping of volcanic rock that extended into the ocean about the length of half a football field. To get a better look at the Nā Pali coastline, I decided to walk out to where hardened lava met ocean. When I reached the end of the lava shoal, I was amazed to see that directly beneath me was a vast coral reef teeming with life. The crystal-clear waters enabled me to see huge schools of fish huddled together, darting back and forth trying to avoid larger fish, maybe the length of your arm. I was immediately consumed with my boyish obsession for fishing, fantasizing about what kind of fish I might be able to pull from the depths.

I had definitely overpacked for this trip, in an attempt not to be underequipped for whatever excursion I decided to take upon my arrival. My procrastination of unpacking the car last night definitely paid off today, because I remembered that still in the trunk was my rod, reel, and tackle. I excitedly hopped from one rock to the next all the way back to the beach and to the car to retrieve my fishing gear.

Now, I didn't know if I needed a permit or a license to fish here, but at the time it didn't matter to me; I was now on a mission. If I got caught, it would be well worth the fine, and I would not be keeping whatever I caught, anyway; I always catch and release. So once I had my gear, again I jumped from rock to craggy rock, bursting with excitement to get my line in the water. I once again got to the end of the lava outcrop and quickly sifted through my tackle box for what to use. I had noticed previously the larger fish were chasing smaller, bait-sized fish, so I put on a silvery spoon lure that imitated a minnow.

I must have cast for an hour, trying all different kinds of lures and setups. Slow retrievals, jerking motions, whatever I could think of, but no luck. I guess my years of fishing for bass and trout just didn't translate into fishing on a coral reef. Once again I was fumbling through my tackle box when I happened to notice beneath me, in a large crevice, a small crab turned upside down and motionless. He must have gotten upended by a crashing wave and gotten stuck there when the tide went out. In any case he wasn't moving, so I got down on my knees and reached for one of his claws. I pulled him up, and he definitely was dead, but it must have been recent, because there was no odor. That's when I got the idea…I grabbed a small broken piece of lava and cracked open his shell. I put a leader on my line now with a hook instead of a lure and put a good quarter-sized piece of crab meat on the end of my line. I cast it just past where the coral reef opened up, hoping real bait might trump artificial lures.

Sure enough, not ten seconds after that crab hit the water, wham! Something hit the bait hard and started to run. I set the drag, and the fight was on, my heart pounding in my chest. I had absolutely no idea, if whatever I had hooked didn't break my line, what I was going to pull out of this ocean. As I felt him tire, and I was able to slowly reel him in, my excitement grew, fixated on what might be on the end of my hook. As I continued to pull him up from the depths and now above the reef, I could now see his dark silhouette, highlighted by the lighter coral. His outline was smaller than I had imagined him being, based on the fight he put up, and as I got him near the surface, he made one last attempt to dive. I pulled up on the rod tip, stopping his retreat, and finally pulled him right out of the Pacific.

I was amazed at what I saw as I placed him next to me on the ledge. The fish was about two feet long and was a rainbow of pastel colors, glistening in the sun. His mouth looked like a bird's beak, obviously adapted to pecking at the coral. Being an avid saltwater-aquarium enthusiast, I immediately recognized him as a parrot fish. Only in my aquarium, he was the size of your finger, not the size of your leg like this one. He flopped around a couple of times, so I grabbed him firmly around his belly as I easily removed the hook. I quickly approached the water, fish cradled in my arms, and placed him back in the ocean. With a quick flick of the tail, he was gone. I just stood there, basking in the shock over what I had just caught. That lasted about three seconds before I ran back to the crab, baited my hook again, and threw my line about ten yards to the left of where I had just cast.

Wham! Again, in ten seconds, I had another hard strike, and immediately I set the hook. I could tell right away this was a different species, as the fight was much different, this time much more aggressively pulling, like a steelhead trout. Once again I got him to the surface, and I pulled from the Pacific another gigantic version of a fish that I had in my aquarium at home. This time it was a Niger trigger...a very aggressive species of fish, so beautiful in color and shape that his cousin is named the Picasso triggerfish.

As I once again picked the fish up and prepared to remove the hook, I was startled by a voice from behind me..."Are you going to keep him?"

I spun around in surprise to see before me a very dark-complexioned, quite obviously native islander in what looked to be only a loincloth.

"Ummm…no" was the only thing I could manage to get to leave my lips.

"Well, may I, then?" he requested.

I removed the hook and held him out, while he was still squirming in my clutches. The native grabbed him from me by the gills with one hand and turned around back toward the beach. I watched his retreat all the way past the shore and eventually to the line of palms. He sat down there on a towel, next to what looked like a lean-to fashioned from bamboo and palm leaves. He had a small makeshift fire pit next to his shelter, and from this distance he looked as if he started to clean the fish I had just provided him.

Now feeling like I was encroaching on an indigenous person's claim of property, I quickly packed up my gear and made my way to the beach. He must have been watching me too, because he was walking toward me now with something in his hands. As we approached one another, he held out a pair of fresh coconuts and exclaimed, *"No ka i'a!"*

I nodded, smiled, and said, *"Mahalo,"* as he handed me the coconuts. It was the only word I actually knew, and it had come in handy that day. I continued to sit in my car watching him, fascinated by the person I had just met. I went back out on the beach, sitting in the sand, trying not to make it too obvious that he was intriguing to me. A couple of hours passed, and he walked back out to the ocean and dived in. I lost sight of him for a couple of moments, but then he resurfaced, took a deep breath, and seemed to dive deep. After about a minute, I stood up, trying to get a glimpse of where he had gone, focusing on where I thought I saw him descend. Out of the corner of my eye, and about twenty yards away from where I was staring, I saw a huge crab pop out of the surf. Holding the crab with one hand, and swimming back with the other, the native made his way back to shore. He nodded at me as he made his way back to his bamboo lean-to.

I fantasized for a moment, wondering what it might be like to just forget all my worldly possessions and live on the beach, partaking of the ocean's bounty whenever I felt the pang of hunger, living sort of like Tom Hanks's character in the movie *Cast Away*, the one exception being the public restrooms, of course. That moment was fleeting, as I looked down at my smartphone, waved good-bye to the native, and hopped in my rental Jeep to head back to the hotel and Egyptian cotton sheets.

3.3 KALALAU

The next day's planned activity was something I had circled on the calendar and looked forward to for a long time: hiking the Kalalau Trail on the Nā Pali Coast. Google activities in Kauai, and this trail always tops the list, and for good reason. If you have ever been on the Pacific Coast Highway in California, it boasts some of the most spectacular views the North American continent has to offer as it parallels and winds its way around the Pacific coastline. This trail basically does the same thing, only on foot, and with all due respect to Californians; California State Route 1 pales in comparison.

The day started with packing up my backpack; this hike was going to include an overnight at the campsite at the end of the trail. This hike has a reputation for being pretty rigorous, so the pack weighed in at close to thirty-five pounds, with bladders full of water and enough food to last the full two days. As I mentioned earlier, the trailhead starts from the same beach where I had made the new native friend the day before. So once I had everything secured in the backpack, I loaded up and drove back to Ke'e Beach. Upon my arrival I took a quick scan of the beach, but to my dismay, my new friend had obviously packed up and moved on.

Eager to get started on the day's hike, I grabbed my backpack and headed toward the trailhead. As you enter the Kalalau Trail, you are immediately met with an uphill climb into the rain forest. A spider web of roots from the fig trees that line the trail made the initial climb a little more interesting. As I got deeper into the forest, and surrounded by the lush foliage, it was easy to see why this had been the setting for the filming of *Jurassic Park*. It wasn't long before the climb leveled, and I could see glimpses of the ocean through the dense forest. Then all of a sudden, the trail opened up, and I was greeted with a cool breeze off the ocean and a view I would not soon forget.

The Nā Pali Coast, in all its splendor, consists of huge, sheer volcanic cliffs covered in lush greenery that dive straight down into the crystal-blue waters of the Pacific. From this vantage point, you can see a sliver of one of the only beaches on the Nā Pali Coast that is accessible by foot. Hanakapiai Beach is world renowned for both its spectacular beauty and its extremely dangerous riptides. I was now only about a mile hike from the beach's shore as the trail dived back into the forest and descended into the Hanakapiai valley. The vast amount of rainwater traveling down the side of the valley form numerous streams that you need to navigate with caution. Depending on the rain that day, the streams can get swollen very quickly with fast-moving rapids. Many people have needed rescue from this very spot.

As I neared the two-mile mark of the eleven-mile hike, the heat and humidity of the rain forest, combined with the weight of the backpack, started to take its toll…so as I carefully traversed the last stream, I was delighted to see the trail opening up to Hanakapiai Beach. The much-acclaimed beauty of this beach cannot be over-exaggerated, and it would prove the perfect setting for me to rest up while admiring the scenery. As I approached a sheltered area of the beach, far removed from the hot rays of the sun, I couldn't help but notice a sign that someone obviously had handmade while telling an ominous tale: "DO NOT GO NEAR THE WATER. UNSEEN CURRENTS HAVE KILLED!" And then beneath that were scratches scribed into the sign, much as soldiers did, marking their kills on rifles in World War II. These scratches commemorated the number of souls who had not heeded the warnings and had ventured out into the ocean. I counted eighty-two marks scribed into that old wooden sign, and I did not intend to be number eighty-three that day.

Once I had rehydrated and had a snack, I was back on my way. The trail ascended once more onto the cliff face of the Nā Pali coastline and then back once again into the rain forest. It alternated like that for the next couple of miles; one minute you were crossing a stream, the next you were gazing out onto the ocean. At mile marker six, you descend down into the Hanakoa valley; this would basically be the halfway point. Once you reach the campsite at the base of the valley, you are rewarded with an awe-inspiring view of a waterfall at the peak of one of the multitude of mountains, shedding a huge volume of tropical rainfall. I was pretty well spent at that point and decided to rest there for about an hour to get reenergized for the hairiest portion of the trail that lay just ahead. It started to drizzle now, and a mist had settled in…like I said, the wettest place on the planet.

The rainfall was a little disconcerting now, knowing what part of the trail I was about to navigate. The trail now opened back up onto the ocean, and the northern cliffs of the Nā Pali coastline were in full view. From this vantage point, you could see exactly what the next quarter mile of trail had in store for you.

It is justly referred to as Crawler's Edge…and that is not an embellished description; it is literally how you have to spend the next few hundred yards. This portion of the hike circumnavigates one of the sheer volcanic cliffs, starting first with a decent-sized trail and then narrowing down to the width of your shoe. The wet and slippery conditions now only enhanced the perilous nature of how I would spend the next fifteen minutes. I suggest searching the Internet for Crawler's Edge videos, because I cannot begin to describe how precarious it felt being halfway up on a sheer volcanic cliff, the ocean menacingly crashing 150 feet below your feet. Numerous people have lost their lives on this stretch of "trail," including one Japanese tourist who was allegedly pushed.

Once I confirmed there was not another soul behind me or in front of me whom I would then have to try to step around to get past, I embarked on the scariest three hundred yards of my life. Let me preface this by saying I have always had a significant fear of heights that I am sure I inherited from my father. I definitely didn't have it as bad as he did, though, as he once made us sit on a train for three days in order to go to my sister's wedding in California, but it still ranks right up there on the short list of things that give me the most anxiety.

So I grabbed a handful of rock in my left hand to steady myself, and off I went. Trying not to get a glimpse of the ocean below, I turned and faced the cliff as I shimmied down the now rain-soaked path, all the while holding on to one craggy volcanic rock after the next for support. Seconds felt like hours as I stepped sideways with my right foot and then met it with the left. Once I got about midway, I came to a particularly hazardous section where there was really no longer any sign of a trail at all. I froze there for a minute as I inadvertently caught a peek of the Pacific crashing beneath…and then I felt that wave of anxiety start to creep in. This definitely wasn't the first time I had faced this rush of apprehension, and with what I was likely going to face down the road in my life, it damn sure wasn't going to be the last…so I took a deep, long breath, shut my eyes, and pictured the one person who gives me the most joy and inner peace in my life…my daughter, Gracie. There have always been a few specific memories that we've shared that I am able to recount and focus on during these trying times that give me solace. Etched in my mind is holding her tiny little hand in my own as she lay beside me, taking long, deep breaths in peaceful slumber. Getting her dressed up as a princess right before our tour of Disneyworld is another of my favorite comforting mental pictures. But likely the most vivid, as well as being the most soothing, would be recalling the look of delight on her face as she took her very first few steps across the kitchen floor and into my arms. So whatever it might be for you…that one specific person who inspires calm, a previous vacation on a beach, or even a starry, tranquil night…I would highly encourage having that one go-to image that inspires serenity and relaxation. I have found it to be life-saving.

With my composure regained, I carefully navigated those next few precarious yards, first testing the footing before transferring all my weight. Within the next few minutes, I was past the worst of it, the trail widened, and I was home free. The remaining four miles were basically the same as the previous six, alternating from rain forest to coastline, and eventually I made it to my final destination for the night, Kalalau Beach. At that point I was physically and mentally exhausted and labored to set up my tent at the campsite. I slept like a log, and the next day I was up early and hiked the same trail back. Having already been across it once, Crawler's Edge posed far less peril this time around, not to mention it was dry as a bone. I cut about an hour off my previous day's hike, and by three o'clock I was on my way back to Princeville.

The following day was my last in Kauai, so I planned what I thought would be a nice, leisurely day to enjoy the last bit of the Nā Pali Coast land-scape and, if I had the energy, maybe even some of its aquatic splendor. To that end, I booked a boat excursion that takes you around the most scenic side of the Nā Pali Coast, as the terrain is much too formidable to even consider building a road. I had a relaxing morning and started on my way to the launch site on the north end of Kauai, at Hanalei Bay. I met our captain for the day and was introduced to three couples who would be joining us for the trip. These boat tours are pretty much all-inclusive, supplying snacks, Gatorade, and even the snorkeling equipment. The plan was to leave from Hanalei Bay and end up in Turtle Bay on the northwest side of the Nā Pali Coast, which has an amazing coral reef. On the way we would spot pods of dolphins or whales and explore the many sea caves, carved over the millennia, from waves crashing into the cliffs.

The excursion started out on fairly calm seas, but once we left the relative shelter of the bay, large rolling waves kept the captain on his toes. For anyone who is a boat enthusiast, we were in a center-console-style Zodiac that was about twenty-eight feet in length. It was smaller than most, but that was advantageous for navigating the caves.

We had been moving at a pretty good clip, well into a half an hour, when the captain cut the motor and pointed to about twenty yards off the bow. A pod of dolphins was vigorously circling a huge school of baitfish they had corralled, the ocean surface now frothing from the smaller fishes' feverish yet fruitless attempts at escape. The dolphins seemed to be a big reason why most of the people in our party had booked this trip, so we stayed for about a half hour, admiring the dolphins' ingenuity.

We motored away once the dolphins had had their fill, heading back toward the coastline and the sea caves. The fifteen-minute trip to the caves flew by as we all sat back admiring the majestic coast with the backdrop of the clear and intensely blue sky. As we approached the first cave, the captain maneuvered the boat with masterful precision, clearly demonstrating his years of experience. The first cave we entered was somewhat claustrophobic at first but then opened up into a huge cavern, open to the sky, with a huge waterfall gracing its exit and crystal-clear water teeming with fish. It looked as if it were taken directly from a postcard. Once again, words or pictures just don't do this experience justice.

Another thirty minutes passed of the captain adroitly darting in and out of the various sea caves, and then once again we were back out on the open Pacific. We were on our way to the final destination of Turtle Bay, when the captain once again cut the motor. Pointing up at the vast Kauaian landscape, he pronounced, "Up in those mountains, an ancient race of people…the first people on this island, are said to have mysteriously vanished." He went on to explain that according to Hawaiian mythology, there was an early race that inhabited the island before the Polynesians, named the Menhune. According to island lore, this tribe, although much smaller in stature than the average native, were very adept craftspeople. Fish ponds, dams, and even ancient temples had been discovered that predated the Tahitian invasion that occurred in the 1100s. According to legend, when the first Polynesian settlers arrived, they subdued the Menhune, whom they considered an inferior race. The Menhune fled into the mountains, never to be heard from again. On our way to Turtle Bay, we all strained our eyes looking up at the mountains, hoping to see some evidence of a past civilization.

Another twenty-minute ride and we reached our ultimate destination of Turtle Bay, named after the large population of green sea turtles that frequent this abundant feeding ground. Turtle Bay is a massive sheltered cove, whose ocean floor is almost completely covered in a coral reef. There is no beach or road access to this area, and it is only reachable by boat, which made this destination seem that much more exotic. As we arrived, the captain killed the motor and proceeded to point to where he kept the snorkeling equipment. We all grabbed snorkels, fins, and masks, only to hear from the captain, "There are no shark warnings for this area today, so have a great time." Immediately one of the women put her snorkel back in the storage compartment. I was feeling fairly rested, so I decided to don a mask and hop overboard for a minute to see if I wanted to put on the rest of the gear.

To have referred to this reef as one of the wonders of the world would not have been an overstatement. It was absolutely bursting with sea life, like I had just jumped into a colossal saltwater aquarium. I hurriedly climbed up the swim ladder and back into the boat, excitedly attempting to convince everyone who hadn't picked up a mask to do so ASAP. Sharks or no sharks, there was nothing stopping me from going in now, so I grabbed a snorkel and fins and returned to explore the reef.

The colors and the clarity were more vivid than you can imagine. I immediately saw the parrot fish I'd had on the end of my line a few days earlier, pecking at the living coral just like I had imagined it would. Swimming past him, I came upon a school of brilliantly colored yellow tang and butterfly angelfish. I was just amazed at the sheer size of everything…small fist-sized urchins you would see at a pet store were the size of basketballs. As I skimmed the surface of the reef, enchanted by this entire ecosystem, I saw a large object swim by in my peripheral. I thought it was another snorkeler, but to my surprise and delight, it was a huge green sea turtle. I immediately turned to follow her and noticed a smaller baby sea turtle swimming about three feet beneath her. As I followed I felt I was witnessing something pretty rare, or at least out of the ordinary, because I had always read that sea turtles abandoned their young to fend for themselves. In any case I wasn't letting them out of my sight. We swam together in and out of the coral, circling around, and at one point the big turtle came close enough for me to touch. Surprisingly, she wasn't startled in the least. I was hovering over the turtles as they swam, my swim fins enabling me to keep up to their pace. On the next such occasion, when she rose close to the surface, I latched onto the back of her shell. Not showing a hint of fear, she let me ride along for a good thirty seconds before diving back down about ten yards deep. I continued to shadow them from above, mesmerized by this interaction.

This went on about three or four more times until I finally lost them in the depths. It was probably a good thing, because I felt like I was really beginning to feel drained, most likely from the previous day's hike. I popped my head up to see in which direction I needed to swim to get back in the boat.

To this day, I have never been as horrified as I was in that moment. Where was the boat? I spun around frantically looking for it and was absolutely aghast to see that the boat was now no bigger than my fist on the horizon line. But that wasn't even the worst part, as I heard a thunderous crash behind me. As I turned around, I realized that somehow I was now only about thirty yards away from being chopped to bits by the ten-foot waves pounding into the black razor-sharp volcanic cliffs behind me. I realized in that moment that I had gotten so caught up in following those goddamn turtles that I lost all track of time and my location. As I got nearer to the coastline, I must have gotten swept up into some sort of a current that had now placed me less than half a football field away from my certain demise. I frantically scoured the cliff line for some sort of shore I could possibly swim to, but there wasn't one for as far as the eye could see in either direction.

Panic started to set in...I knew full well if I allowed that to happen, I was done for. You see, my mother had been a lifeguard the majority of her adult life, and she insisted that her kids get certified as such too. I heard her in my head now, what she had taught me from a very early age. "You panic in the water, and you're dead."

She taught me to put my head back, breathe deeply, and tread water until I could calm myself down. I had learned this twenty-five years earlier, yet it came back to me as if it was instinct, as if she was whispering it into my ear.

I flipped my mask up, put my head back, and started to tread water. In probably about thirty seconds of performing this technique, I had a calm come over me that to this day still comforts me. It was as if I accepted that I was going to die, and all the fear drained from my body. Now don't get me wrong; my will to live was still there, and I was going to fight like hell for my survival, but I knew in that moment, if I died everything would be OK. Call it your brain's reaction for self-preservation, call it divine intervention, how-ever your set of beliefs decide to classify it, the acceptance of death saved my life.

Then I heard my mom's voice again, "*Now swim!*"

I ripped the mask off, and just as I turned around, readying myself to swim toward the boat, a huge wave crashed down upon me, filling my lungs. As I was slammed deep by the incred-ible force of the wave, I thought, *This is it. Game over...*but somehow I bobbed back up to the sur-face, not yet close enough to be thrown into the rocks. I hacked and coughed up the wretched salt water. Once I got my bearings, I again treaded water with my head back, and after three long breaths, I pointed myself in the direction of the boat and just did as my mom had instructed; I started swimming. The flippers gave me enough of an extra thrust to counteract the current. If I had lost them when the wave hit me, I wouldn't be writing this. I swam for what seemed like hours, but it probably was more like twenty min-utes...and luckily for me, at this point the captain had been scouring the surface of the water with binoculars, looking for me. I remember looking up one last time and seeing the boat, now much closer, speeding toward me. At that point I was completely and utterly drained. I strained to lift my arm another stroke. The last thing I remember is being dragged up into the boat, completely limp and barely able to move a muscle.

Chapter 4

4.1 TANZANIA

As our prop plane buzzed the grass airstrip at the Selous Game Reserve in southern Tanzania, I quickly realized how close I was to no longer being on the top of the food chain. Banking a hard left, the pilot, now satisfied there were no elephants or large herds of wildebeest to impede our landing, leveled for our final descent. This was the land bordered by Kenya, Uganda, and the Congo—with the Indian Ocean to the east and Mount Kilimanjaro's peak to the north. In the air, and from this vantage point, there were a countless array of rivers and streams, almost resembling the underside of a maple leaf from a childhood science project. Fed by the *masika* (Swahili for rainy season), these rivers stretched for miles in all directions and sustained life for its indigenous creatures, as well as took life by camouflaging its predators in their shadowy depths. As we got closer to touchdown, I noticed how well adapted even the trees had to be in this hostile environment. The flat-topped acacia has even evolved to having no branches or leaves for the first few meters from its base, not to mention very tough bark to ward off grazing beasts and the ever-frequent savannah wildfires.

As the Cessna thumped down and rolled to a stop on one of the roughest patches of the strip, an impala pranced out of the bush about one hundred meters in front of us and turned to give us that startled look I am so used to seeing on its distant cousin, the white-tailed deer. As I opened the door to exit the plane, I was instantly met by a rush of heat and humidity along with a unique smell of death that I have yet to be able to adequately put into words. In that moment I realized I was no longer the king of my domain, like I used to be, while walking on a northern Michigan hiking trail trying to find a good spot to cast for trout. No…now I was much more like that impala, with a sense of fear and extremely heightened senses, wondering what was lurking in the long, tall grass. The glaring difference, however, was that I had neither the speed nor the agility that gave the impala at least a fifty-fifty chance…and as I warily and clumsily walked my way down the airstrip toward the awaiting guide, I realized I much more resembled a wounded animal to anyone or anything that may have been watching.

Maybe I'm getting a little ahead of myself. Let me back up a bit. On this trip, as I've done with all my others, I investigated what I really wanted to get out of this excursion to the African continent and how I could have the best experience possible. We were always mesmerized as kids watching on TV, or reading through the latest *National Geographic*, by the daily life-and-death struggle of the world's most savage predators.

Now every day we get up, have a cup of coffee, check our phones, and get visibly upset over the ranking of our favorite Big 10 team dropping by three spots or what Kim Kardashian dared to reveal in her latest tweet. Did Cadillac just put hand warmers in the steering wheels, and did Burger King just come out with a triple whopper?

For the most part, a civilized human being now has been conditioned to never wonder what it feels like to be thirsty or where the next meal is coming from, let alone wondering if that next meal is going to be you. So this is what brought me to Tanzania...never experiencing those most primitive needs and primal fears meant that I could never truly appreciate the comforts we all enjoy but have never really earned ourselves.

This level of self-fulfillment was not going to be achieved by riding through the Serengeti in a raised and well-protected Jeep, nor by staying in the African version of a five-star resort with hot tubs and Chardonnay. No, the odds needed to be much more even, which is why I chose what is known as a fly-camping expedition.

Fly-camping is basically just that...camping on the fly. Hiking the animal trails during the day and pitching a tent near some of the more tra-versed areas of the nocturnal creatures at night, watering holes and riverbanks primarily. This was going to be a four-day, three-night excursion, and once again, I don't have a death wish; I would have an armed guide with me the whole time... which basically leads me back to where this chap-ter began.

So I flew from Chicago to Amsterdam and then to Kilimanjaro and finally to Dar es Salaam airport. Sixteen long hours later, I'm finally walking on a grass airstrip, clumsily making my way from the plane toward the awaiting guide, carrying two large duffel bags and a big bottle of water. I never gave it much thought, but as the pilot escorted me toward the awaiting guide, I suddenly realized he wasn't going to be the Australian with the hat and thick outback accent whom I had pictured in my head...not even close. From a distance, I realized he looked more like a Zulu tribesman than Crocodile Dundee. As we got nearer, I asked the pilot in a hushed and hopeful tone, "I hope the guide speaks good English?" and the pilot replied, "Oh, you'll see..."

As we approached, the pilot blurted out, "Mr. Scott, meet your guide for the next few days; his name is Adnan."

There was a long, awkward pause while Adnan appeared to be quietly judging my choice of safari gear and trail readiness.

After looking me up and down, Adnan turned toward the pilot and said in surprisingly good English, "Well, he's not in Kansas anymore."

We all laughed out loud. I realized in that moment that I really had never heard myself fake laugh like that before...I mean while simultaneously shitting my pants, that is.

We said our good-byes to the pilot, and Adnan pointed over to an awaiting Jeep with a driver. He made it clear that it was going to be dark soon and that we needed to get to the campsite so we had enough daylight to pitch our tents. We piled my bags in the Jeep and took off down the path where there once seemed to be tire tracks. I watched helplessly as the pilot, and my only link to civilization, buzzed over our heads and waved the airplane's wings in what I thought might be a final farewell. Adnan must have seen the anxiety on my face and labored to find the words that he must have thought might soothe my mind. "Don't you worry; if you need medical attention, he can be back in eight or nine hours." That just made everything seem so much worse.

I remained quiet for the ten-minute drive to camp...partially because I was taking in the scenery, but mostly because I didn't want any more alarming reassurances.

We must have only driven about two miles at most, down a heavily rutted trail that looked more like a tractor path than an actual road, the Jeep finally lurching to a stop at an elevated clearing. Below us was a small cliff perched just above a large watering hole. Adnan and the driver jumped out, quickly throwing both my two large duffel bags on the ground, along with an additional smaller bag, a machete, and what I assumed to be a large-caliber rifle case. Adnan looked at my bags and then gave me another long stare. "Do you intend on carrying both those bags all day tomorrow?"

I sheepishly looked down and shook my head like a punished schoolboy and asked if the driver could please take most of it with him and said that I was sorry for not following the directions more carefully on weight restrictions…

The driver handed me a small backpack as Adnan instructed, "Only what you need for the next three days." I hurried through both my bags and left the majority behind in the back seat. As the driver started the Jeep, a slow, sinking feeling crept into my stomach. I realized I was now being left here alone with an African tribesman, whom I had just met ten minutes ago, while being surrounded by the deadliest predators on the planet…not to mention now it was getting dark.

My vivid imagination, fueled by fear, started going through all the possibilities while I gathered my belongings. I stared at Adnan while gathering my stuff, trying to look for some sort of expression on his face that might give me an indication of what his next move might be. *What is stopping him from just walking off and leaving me here? They have my money already...*His gaze looked somewhat sinister to me now as he surveyed the landscape and again looked in my direction. Maybe he would cut me open with that machete and just wait for the hyenas to get a scent of my blood, devouring me while I was still alive...and then I'd be picked clean by the vultures in the morning. Or maybe he'd just march me right down to the watering hole that was now only fifty yards away...and throw me into the crocodile-infested pool of death where even my bones would be digested, along with every evidence of my existence.

Now he started walking toward me, and that sinister expression now seemed to be more bloodthirsty...I started backing up as he reached into his inner coat pocket. He must have been concealing another smaller handgun or hunting knife; my retreat now gained a little more momentum. Just as I was about to turn and run, my foot sank into one of the deep rutted tire tracks, and I went down hard. Now I was on my back, still pushing away through the tall grass with my legs, fixated on what he was about to pull out of his jacket, as he now was only a couple of feet away. As he approached quickly and now stood over me, I instinctively shielded my face with my arms as he pulled out what I was sure he was going to plunge deep into my chest…"Mr. Scott, would you like this Twinkie before we set up the tent?"

I guess it goes without saying…fear and delusion were now replaced with utter embarrassment. I had once again done what I had come here never to do again: let my surroundings and anxiety get the best of me. Whether it was here at dusk in the African savannah or in a hospital bed only a few miles from my home, I no longer had any patience for these feelings determining my actions or my frame of mind…so I got up, ate that Twinkie, and started to help get camp set up.

4.2 TENTS

With a renewed sense of confidence and a belly full of cream filling, I grabbed one of the small, pillow-case-sized bags that Adnan had pointed to, and pulled out its entire contents. At first glance, it appeared to be about two big handfuls of mosquito netting, so I asked Adnan, "Is this what goes over the tent?"

It was getting dark now, so Adnan shined his flashlight to illuminate what I had bunched up in my hands.

"No...that *is* your tent, and don't worry; we will not be getting any rain tonight. Now please bring that over here; we don't have much time."

I ran the netting over to Adnan, while thinking the whole time that getting wet was the least of my concerns. What could this flimsy netting protect us from? There were more than just little insects thirsting for our blood around here. Adnan had now pounded a series of four poles in the ground, and we draped the first net into place between the poles, stretching them tight. After pounding in another two poles, we finished by draping the second net over them and spiking the ends in the ground. Now basically we had two mosquito-free cubes that were as big as small closets, side by side and joined together by the two inner poles. Adnan grabbed another of the duffel bags the driver had tossed on the ground, from which he then removed a couple of thick rolled-up floor mats and sleeping bags. Once we got our new "beds" rolled out, Adnan lit a lamp and set up two foldaway canvas chairs outside the tents, pointing them in the direction of the watering hole, almost like you would if you were planning to watch your kid's soccer game.

Adnan gestured toward the chairs to sit down. I decided to accept his invitation, as it had been a very long trip, and by now I was convinced I didn't have to keep an eye on his every move for fear of him murdering me.

As I sat, I was immediately struck by how brilliant the stars were in southern Africa, far away from any ambient city lighting. The moon was full now, and it glimmered off the watering hole, lighting up our raised campsite as if we were on a stage in a school play.

"You must be exhausted and thirsty," Adnan asserted as he sat down next to me and offered a canteen of water. As I took a sip and pointed toward the watering hole, I explained that adrenaline and not knowing what was in or around that water was primarily keeping me awake.

"They are not interested in you or me...they are only interested in food and drink."

So I inquired whether this was a popular place to witness nocturnal activity, knowing full well I had seen a lot of movement already down by the water's edge.

"We will see; I have never been here before," Adnan replied with a smirk and a loud chuckle.

Trying not to show how alarmed I was, I politely excused myself by telling Adnan that I really thought I should try to get some sleep so I would be fresh for the next day's hike. And with that I turned around, unzipped the netting to my bedroom, jumped into my bed, and zipped the sleeping bag closed over my head.

I lay there for about an hour pretending to sleep, mostly listening to Adnan shuffling about the camp humming and singing to himself in what must have been his native tongue. A little later, the welcoming sound of crickets chimed in, filling the air with a familiarity, making me feel as comfortable as I had been on the trip so far. It brought back the same feelings and memories of sleeping under the stars in the backyard with my little sister, Julie, hunting for the Big Dipper and catching earthworms in the summer dew. I felt relaxed enough that I finally was able to feel the tightness leave my arms. My neck and back seemed to exhale as the weight of the day had finally taken its toll. My eyelids now heavy, my anxieties surrendering to fatigue, my breathing now deepened as I started to doze off…

I thought it was thunder that woke me up. Startled, I jumped straight up…only now I couldn't figure out where I was, why it was pitch black, and what the hell I was doing tied up and feeling as if I were being smothered! My head was spinning, such as it does when you are awoken from a bad dream. Now I was gasping for air, figuring that maybe I only had a few breaths left before I ran out of oxygen. Was it a dream? Had I been buried alive? As my wits started to return, remembering where I was and how I had fallen asleep, I realized I was still inside my sleeping bag…having zipped it shut over my head. As I struggled to find the zipper, I got another sample of what had just awoken me from a dead sleep in the first place.

The sound first registers in your ears as would a loud clap of thunder, rapidly grabbing your attention. But then immediately it resonates through your bones, as you realize in the pit of your stomach that this is not just some nightmare that you can quickly shake off and wake up from. No, this was a primal and savage roar, alerting every living thing within a mile's radius that the king of all beasts was on the prowl and in your vicinity.

I froze like a statue...on my knees, in my brown sleeping bag still zipped closed over my head.

"Adnan," I whispered loudly. "Adnan!" I listened intently for a few moments, now hyper-focused on my surroundings. I heard what seemed to be a low, rhythmic growl, quiet at first but getting increasingly louder. I strained my ears, trying to identify what it was, and then it dawned it me...it was Adnan snoring!

"Adnan!" I said, much more loudly this time as I crawled on my knees toward where I thought his bed might be, all the while fidgeting with trying to find the zipper so I could extricate my head from this sleeping bag. Just then, another massive roar rang out, and this time it seemed much closer.

I now picked up my pace, scurrying on my knees, and this time screamed out, "Adnan, wake up!"

I then was knocked to the ground by what seemed like something similar to a metal flashlight hitting me on top of the head. I turned over on my back, and the zipper on my sleeping bag started opening up to reveal Adnan's face peering down at me.

"You know you collapsed both of our tents, right, man? Help me put the poles back up."

I quickly scurried out of my sleeping bag and asked if he had his gun.

"I told you, they are not interested in me or you," he said as he pointed down to the watering hole.

As I turned and grabbed a breath, I quickly counted one large male lion and four females lying down at the water's edge, lazily lapping up some water and basking in the moon's silvery glow.

"Like I said before, they are only interested in food or drink," Adnan said in obvious frustration. "Now can you please help me set our tents up again?"

Once the tents were back up, I brought one of the chairs inside the netting, and the rest of that night I stared down at the watering hole. I was entranced watching the reflection of the smaller animals darting to and fro, attempting to get just a sip of water while trying to avoid certain death. That night I heard some of the most bone-chilling and blood-curdling sounds that no audio recording is capable of replicating, not to mention the sounds of Adnan's blissful slumber.

I was grateful to see the sun rising above the horizon. As the mist rose from the water, the birds started chirping, and thankfully the man-eaters commenced their exit. I finally felt safe enough to go to sleep for about thirty minutes before Adnan awoke.

"Come, Mr. Scott," Adnan urged while shaking my foot to awaken me. "Eat a quick breakfast bar; we have a good long hike in front of us."

I mustered up what energy I had left to start packing what little gear remained in my possession. The sun at this point had already crept its way well up into the morning sky, my loose-fitting long-sleeve T-shirt quickly starting to dampen from the stagnant heat and swamp-like humidity.

We each wolfed down a protein bar, surveyed the area for any remnants of the night's excitement, and made our way toward what I would loosely call a path. The hike that morning consisted mostly of me swatting at large tsetse flies and asking Adnan to elaborate about his life. Adnan seemed pretty shy and reserved about opening up about his personal life; instead, he focused on showing me what might bring me peril if I was not cautious while traipsing through his native land.

Most notably, he veered off the path slightly toward a lone acacia tree and exclaimed, "Mr. Scott, come here quickly! I caught a glimpse of him out of the corner of my eye. They sun themselves in the morning before they hunt."

Never trailing more than a few short steps behind Adnan, I hurried over toward where he had come to a complete halt. I thought Adnan might be pointing to a baby lemur or maybe even an anteater, which I had researched as being another tree dweller in Africa…I wasn't even close.

I stopped a couple of feet short when I realized what Adnan was trying to show me. Stretched among four of five lower limbs was a long olive-colored snake, and he did not look overly pleased at our presence. He had gone from lying down flat and soaking up the morning sun to adopting an aggressive, cobra-like stance while still in the tree. Once he took that position, and I got a better look at his head, I backed up even farther.

"Adnan, is that a mamba?" I timidly asked while retreating still.

"Yes," he replied, "a black mamba. You can tell by the inside of his mouth." He waved his machete at him in order to initiate a harmless strike. "I wanted to show you what they look like and where they nest. They are much more dangerous than your lion friend last night." And at that the black mamba quickly slithered down the tree and sped away in the opposite direction from where I was standing.

"You do not want to come near him," Adnan warned once again. "I was once in class with a younger man who looked a lot like you. We were both in school to become safari guides here on the savanna. One day we were hiking a trail very near the school, and we came across a nest with a much smaller black mamba. My friend, the young student, was overly eager to impress our teacher with the skills he had recently learned regarding handling serpents. The mamba reared up, just like this one did in the tree a few minutes ago. The snake lunged for my friend and, we thought, nearly bit him, and then it fled. About thirty minutes later, my friend collapsed and fell unconscious. We took him to hospital, but it was too late; he died on the table. They found a very tiny mark on his leg where he had gotten a small bite. Their venom can kill one hundred men... please just go the other way if you see one."

Adnan didn't need to warn me about black mambas. I already had researched them pretty thoroughly before I got to the continent, finding out that more people are killed on safari by them than by any of the other large predators combined. Not only are they easily agitated, but they are one of if not *the* fastest snakes in existence. On top of that, and if they weren't already frightening enough, they can raise themselves up sometimes as much as four to five feet off the ground and nearly look you right in the eye before filling you full of deadly venom.

I caught back up to Adnan once I was sure the mamba was long gone in the other direction.

We continued our hike in the heat of the day, stopping briefly at times for Adnan to point out a distant elephant or herd of zebra. We came upon a lone rhinoceros about two hundred yards away, and that's when Adnan made the first inquiry of me. "Mr. Scott, people I guide who are not hunters are usually taking hundreds of photos each day and making me pose with them every fifteen minutes. Yet you don't bring a phone and have not taken a single picture…what is your reason?"

I smiled and nodded my head. "I get that question a lot, Adnan. People around me are obsessed with documenting every minute of their lives with photos and videos. I am of the opposite mind-set. I don't believe you can authentically experience the moment if you are worried about how that memory will be framed. Of course, I will take a few pictures, but I don't want it to spoil my adventure."

We spent the next couple of hours tracking a course along a trail that was frequented by some of the larger animals in the area. We happened upon a few wildebeest languidly making their way from one patch of tall grass to the next, but not much else for the next couple of hours. I was thankful for the respite, as it gave me an opportunity to learn a bit more about a culture and a man who had become thoroughly intriguing to me. It turned out that Adnan wasn't even close to what one might gather at first appearance. He was nowhere near a bloodthirsty poacher posing as an African guide. Quite the contrary…

Adnan's roots are with the Sukuma tribe of Tanzania. Their name, "Sukuma," literally means "north," simply because most of his five million people live in northern Tanzania. Adnan speaks both Sukuma (Bantu) and English, and like the majority of the Tanzanian Sukuma, Adnan's father was a farmer and raised cattle. His father earned enough money farming to send Adnan to a Jesuit school, where he was taught Christianity and English. Unlike his other seven brothers and sisters, who, like the majority of the Sukuma tribespeople, still believe in and pray to different spirits and gods, Adnan was converted to Christianity at a young age. He graduated with the equivalent of our middle-school education. He decided, instead of following in his father's footsteps of farming, to go into a profession that was responsible for the vast majority of Tanzania's GDP: tourism. His immediate family is still steeped in very traditional Sukuma tribe tradition and culture, whereas Adnan has taken his own path, and his employer provides living quarters for their guides along with free schooling.

"I have told you much about myself...now it is your turn. What are you doing out here by yourself?"

I took a minute to ponder that question. Up until then I had never really expressed to anyone else what I was dealing with from a health standpoint or why I had started to make these life-altering decisions. I guess because I didn't want to burden anyone else with the gravity of what I was dealing with. I'm not sure if it was the heat of the day, the fact that I had just slept less than my driveway's length away from wild predators, or just Adnan's calming and gentle demeanor...but it all came pouring out.

It felt very cathartic in a way to finally get a lot of that baggage off my chest...even if it was to a complete stranger halfway around the world, who may or may not even have understood what I just spent twenty minutes explaining. I was pleasantly surprised with Adnan's reaction and understanding.

"Thank you for your honesty and sharing those very intimate details about your life with me, Mr. Scott...you are very brave."

"I appreciate that, Adnan, and now that we are being completely honest about everything with one another, can I tell you something?"

"Of course," Adnan replied.

"I thought you were going to murder me that first day."

"I still may, Mr. Scott, if you knock down our tent again tonight."

The second night thankfully was much less eventful as we joined our tents in a clearing near the trail we had been following. Adnan's siblings working the cotton fields, my parents raising six kids on a teacher's salary, and even Obama's reelection were all topics of conversation that night. Adnan set up a lamp between our bedrolls so we could at least see what was going on around our immediate vicinity, and I finally passed out from jet lag and utter exhaustion.

The next morning I arose early and paced around camp to see if there had been any activity during the night. Adnan woke up shortly thereafter, stretching with a big yawn, and then handed me another breakfast bar and some juice mix.

4.3 TIGER FISH

We quickly packed up camp and then were on our way to what I considered the highlight of this trip and what I thought would be the most memorable activity of my safari. I mentioned earlier that I had frequented the woods in the Midwest in search of good trout streams. I was never a hunter, but fishing for me was a passion that started at a very young age. My father would take me to catch small bluegill at a local pond around the age of six or seven. That early exposure spawned a passion in me that grew into an obsession. During my early teens, I couldn't buy enough *Field and Stream* magazines to quench my thirst to read about wrestling sixty-pound king salmon out of the famed Kenai River of Alaska during their late July spawning run. Frequently after the bus dropped me off from school, I would throw down my book bag, grab my tackle box, jump on my bike, and ride four miles to the nearest pond. I would cast large popper lures for bass until either my arms felt like they were going to fall off or the sun set…whichever came first. I eventually graduated to fishing for trout and steelhead almost exclusively. They embodied all that I found the most exciting about fishing. Strong, hard-hitting, and very aggressive, they are some of the most thrilling and beautiful fish to battle in North America.

So with that intro, it should come as no surprise…Adnan and I now were only a few minutes' hike away from testing out my angling skills on one of the world's most abundant and hostile rivers on the planet, the Rufiji. The vast Rufiji stretches from the inner African continent almost four hundred miles, before emptying into the mouth of what borders Africa to the east, the Indian Ocean. This historic waterway formerly served as a branch of river ports and commerce for the ancient Greeks and Romans dating back to the first century AD, also allowing archaic merchants to transport the abundance of inland African riches to the open sea.

However, I had not traveled sixteen hours, fending off malaria-transmitting mosquitos and sleeping among Earth's most bloodthirsty predators, for a nice little leisurely and historic boat ride in the late-afternoon sun. No sir, I was here to hunt one of the world's most savage freshwater predators known to man. Growing to an average weight between twenty-five and one hundred pounds of pure streamlined muscle, this highly aggressive fish is closely related to the piranha, but this is no species you would ever want in your aquarium. Named after its land-based equivalent, the tiger fish and its monstrous brother, the goliath tiger fish, exhibit many of the same predatory instincts as their terrestrial namesake. Hunting together only in packs with similarly sized tiger fish, because they would simply devour smaller fish of their own species, they stalk their prey in groups...first rounding them up by encircling their prey in the murky depths and then taking turns maiming them so they cannot flee. This is soon followed by the ferocious pack ripping them to shreds in what can only be aptly described as a rabid feeding frenzy while the water explodes with fury and froth. These are the only fish ever recorded on film jumping out of the water to catch and devour a bird in midflight. If you try to picture a barracuda on steroids, with the mouth of a bear trap, the jaw-clamping strength of a crocodile, and the speed of a dolphin, you will come close to understanding what I desired to latch on to with my fishing pole and a single hook.

Adnan had said the driver was supposed to meet us at the river at four in the afternoon with my fishing gear. When we finally made it to the rendezvous point, the driver had already arrived and was getting my pole equipped with the tackle necessary to land the famed "water devil dog" (as they are referred to by the natives) onto the banks of the Rufiji. The driver handed me the fully equipped fishing pole, and I had to take a minute to fully comprehend what I was looking at. I had never seen such tackle on a fishing pole before, and it was only then that I started to realize what I was actually in store for. At the end of the heavy test fishing line was approximately three feet of thick metal wire with a fastener that clipped to the single barbless hook. This setup was striking, and obviously necessary, due to the combination of the tiger fish's razor-sharp teeth and the violent thrashing that would ensue if I actually hooked into one. Any normal nylon fishing line would be instantly severed.

We gathered up the gear and headed toward the bank of the Rufiji. This time the driver actually joined us, and along with the bait bucket, he carried a large metal spear perched on his right shoulder. Before I could even get the question out, Adnan knew exactly what I was thinking and said, "Just in case the crocs get interested in your fish."

"Ohhh…I see."

As we approached the edge of the river, we seemed to pique the curiosity of some of the resident hippos lounging in the deeper portion of the river. That curiosity quickly subsided once they realized we were just some harmless humans, and even the feathered egrets perched on top of them went back to picking the ticks off the hippos' backs.

Adnan seemed to want to fish right from this spot on the bank, but I suggested we go up the trail a bit where it looked like a nice, calm pool had formed where the river took a sharp bend upstream. As we approached, I was even more encouraged, noticing the shallow rapids that sped up the stream's current and then quickly dumped into the deep pool nestled in the river's inner elbow. Positioned just below that drop-off, in the less turbulent flow of water, was an ideal spot for a large freshwater predator to lie in wait for smaller baitfish to wash through the torrent of the shallow rapids, ultimately plunging into the depths of unknown peril. Based on years of experience, I thought this to be the ideal spot to cast our bait, in an attempt to coax out what I hoped were a pack of these finned hyenas lurking in the shadowy depths, waiting to lunge from beneath for a late-afternoon snack.

I reached for the bucket, which I had instructed Adnan earlier in our trip to fill with large minnows native to the Rufiji, called Kamba minnows. Ranging in size anywhere from eight inches to a foot long, once hooked through the bottom lip, they would squirm and thrash from side to side, making a commotion in the water that was sure to attract the attention of any nearby hunter looking for a quick and easy meal.

So I grabbed one of the Kamba, hooked it through the lip, and cast a bull's-eye into the rapids, landing it just before the deep, circulating pool, at a distance now of about thirty feet from where we stood. Now, in normal circumstances, you would cast a bait where you thought you might have a good shot at a bite and then lock your reel, set your drag, and then comes the long wait. Not in Tanzania, and not in the Rufiji, and definitely not where I had chosen to cast.

As the bait hit the water, I looked down at my reel, and before I could even close the bail, I heard the water explode as if a fat kid had just done a cannonball in front of us...my rod was nearly yanked from my grip as the line started to peel off the open bait casting reel. I instinctively now cranked the reel and jerked back on the pole, knowing that I had to try to tighten the line and bury the hook deep into that bone and teeth-filled mouth to have even a chance of landing whatever had just savagely taken the bait. When I reared the pole back over my head to set the hook, I felt the weight and sheer strength of what had just devoured that poor minnow. This was no five-pound bass; it felt as though another man, stronger than me, was pulling on the end of the line. As the line hissed and screamed as it left my reel, I spun the drag to increase the resistance before I completely ran out of line...the twenty-pound test was leaving my reel more quickly than I had ever witnessed before. I then lowered my fishing-rod tip to take some of the stress off the line, and as I did, the line immediately went limp. I had lost him, and I really was not the least bit surprised. During my research on this type of fishing, I had learned that because of the aggressive nature of this fight, and the armor-like plating in this monster's mouth, only one in ten of these fish ever make it to shore to be netted. As I reeled in my line, now with absolutely no resistance at all, I wondered if I would ever get a second chance at that rush of adrenaline again. As my hook and rig got close to shore, I reeled in the last few turns and raised the tip of the rod to inspect my tackle. I looked over at Adnan in amazement. The only thing left dangling off that hook were the Kamba minnow's lips.

"I guess he won't be needing those anymore." Adnan snickered.

Now I was on a mission. I was landing one of those bastards or would lose a hand trying. I threw the lips in the dirt, grabbed another minnow, and cast into the exact same spot, but this time I was ready. This go-around the bait made it from the shallow rapids into the pool, and it actually sat there for a few seconds, thrashing around from side to side, the sun catching a quick glint off its silvery scales. Had that been my one chance? Did I get lucky enough the first time to cast right in front of the single tiger fish in this part of the river?

Then all of a sudden, the deep pool's serene glass-like surface burst alive again as another fish struck hard, his sheer speed and power now propelling him nearly three feet in the air. We all let out a yell, as there was no mistaking this fish as a fifteen-plus-pound tiger fish, his huge teeth and red fins immediately recognizable as they glistened in the hot afternoon sun. I jerked the tip of the rod up as hard as I could, attempting once again to lodge the hook deep into that bony, prehistoric mouth. This time I felt it sink in deep and solid, and I knew I was in for a battle. The line once again sang from the reel and could only be measured exiting in yards per second, not feet. He swam like a bullet upstream, with me pulling on the rod with every ounce of strength in me, fighting against him burying himself deep underneath the bank of the river, where I would lose him for sure in a tangle of roots and driftwood. As I pulled him back into the relative safety of the depths of the river, the rod bent over so far that I felt like any second it was going to snap in half. Then the rod's bend lessened suddenly, and I would be in a race with him to reel in the line as quickly as humanly possible, as he sped toward me, knowing if I let any slack into the line at all, he would surely throw the hook. The water just in front of us erupted again as the monster tiger burst into the air, shaking his head violently in an attempt to spit out the heavily buried hook. The tiger repeated these runs toward me and then away, probably three more times. I lost count after fighting him for over ten minutes, my heart pounding out of my chest in sheer excitement and utter exhaustion. But now I felt him tiring as well; his runs soon were far less dynamic, and he began to rise to the surface, gasping for air and trying to again shake the hook.

As I slowly reeled him in, now twenty feet away, now fifteen, I slowly felt my excitement mount. I felt I had a real shot at landing this monster as I had dreamed of doing for years. Even Adnan was voicing his approval and grabbed the net to see if I could steer him close enough for him to scoop him up. The tiger now was near the surface, still pulling away and violently shaking his head every few seconds, but I was slowly reeling him in closer to shore.

I got him to about ten feet from the bank, perfectly directing him toward Adnan's waiting net. Then all of a sudden, out of my peripheral vision, I noticed a huge, dark object screaming toward us in the sky, as you would see a car right before it hit you in the middle of an intersection. Again, the water exploded as an enormous gray bird plunged down on top of the tiger, digging its huge talons into him and separating him from my hook. The fish was so big, the eagle (African sea eagle or martial eagle, from what I have since learned) couldn't fly away and actually had to drag him along the surface of the water, landing on the opposite side of the river. I just stood there in amazement…reeling from the fact that you really could never let your guard down for a minute in this environment, or you could end up like that tiger fish or, even worse, that minnow. I glared over at the eagle on the other side of the Rufiji as he now, almost tauntingly, pecked at the fish I had just served up for him on a platter. We all just shook our heads in disbelief.

The sun was now getting a little lower as evening was approaching. I had three more attempts at landing a tiger fish that evening and finally was successful on the third and final attempt. This one was about eight pounds, and up close he was both one of the most beautiful specimens of fish I had ever seen and one of the most horrific. Of course, I released him to live and fight another day (after letting Adnan's driver get the hook out of his mouth). It quite possibly was the most thrilling and adrenaline-filled activity of the trip…well, up to that point, anyway.

As evening grew nearer, we packed up the fishing gear into the Jeep, and the driver was off, leaving us behind with the necessities we needed to make camp for our third and final night. Adnan suggested as a safety measure we go a little farther inland off the river and camp in a place he was familiar with not too far away. After about a twenty-minute hike, we were in a clearing surrounded by a few trees. There was already a fire pit between the trees, and it looked as if it had been used fairly recently. I was sure to get the best sleep of the trip so far, knowing this was a well-traversed campsite. We were losing light rapidly, so we pitched the mosquito tent near one of the trees and built a fire so we could warm up some canned stew that Adnan had on the menu this evening. We sat around the fire in the canvas chairs, and Adnan remarked, "That smile has not left your face since you caught that first fish."

My smile grew thinking back on the day. "I can honestly say, Adnan, that was one of the most amazing experiences I have ever had in my life…thank you."

"I just showed you where the river was," Adnan replied.

We both just smiled now and continued to recount the day's excitement.

The stars once again were ablaze against the stark contrast of the clear black sky, the moon illuminating the savannah, painting the landscape with a soft, consoling glow. I leaned back, basking in the glory of how positively breathtaking it was to be able to experience nature at this most elemental level. I remember thinking in that moment, if my life were to come to an end at this very minute…I could leave this existence satisfied in knowing that for however briefly, I had participated in the miracle of life that Mother Nature had created so abundantly here and everywhere on this unique planet.

I lost track of time indulging my senses, knowing this would be my final night in this extraordinary territory. It must have been after midnight when I finally decided to turn in; Adnan had already been snoring for hours. I unzipped the netting, turned the lamp off, and crawled into my sleeping bag. Feeling an overwhelming sense of warmth and contentment, I fell fast asleep in just a few minutes.

Surprisingly, I awoke in the middle of the night. It was still pitch-black and surprisingly calm, the crickets still chirping their melodic chorus. I lifted my head slightly and looked around a bit to see if I could see if something might have woken me. I didn't see anything, so I put my head back down slowly and started to doze off again…until I heard some movement. Startled a bit, I picked my head up again, this time a little more quickly. After about a minute, I laid my head back down, straining my ears to try to get another sample of what I thought I had heard. Only this time, it wasn't a sound that woke me up. As I started to relax, I closed my eyes, again recollecting the day's events…and then I felt it. Something had brushed up against my leg. I jumped about three feet in the air, reaching for the lamp.

Now on my knees, fumbling for the switch, I turned the dimmer on the lamp all the way up so that now it was like daylight in our tent. I quickly spun around, and what I saw immediately made me freeze in sheer terror. Risen up off the ground and in an aggressive stance, staring me straight in the eyes, was a huge black mamba. With his cobra-like hood fully flared and its enormous black gaping mouth wide open, angrily exposing his vicious fangs, I knew I only had seconds before he struck. He hissed loudly and craned his neck back, and I instinctively lifted my arms to shield my face. I just shut my eyes, bracing for the incredibly painful neurotoxins that were about to be savagely injected into my veins.

All I heard next was a loud yell and a swoosh of air. I dived to the ground and opened my eyes only to see Adnan, machete in hand, standing over my bed with the mamba cut in half, still writhing around on the ground. In stunned silence, I lay there as Adnan finished the job by chopping it up twice more. He turned around, grabbed me by the shirt, and picked me up.

"Did he get you?" Adnan yelled.

"No, I don't think so."

He made me strip and looked me up and down with the lamp.

"I don't see anything," he said.

I just sat there, still in disbelief as Adnan grabbed the lamp and walked around the campsite, ensuring there wasn't more than one. After his inspection, he surmised the snake must have slithered between the netting and the bedding.

"I bet he smelled that fish on you," Adnan theorized.

He tossed his coat over the chair and lit a cigarette. Once I'd had a minute to gather myself, I walked over to him and asked him if I could have a drag.

When we finished his smoke, I walked up to him and gave him a hug. "Oh my God, thank you. You saved my life."

As I stepped back, he looked into my eyes and, with a very serious look on his face, said, "You shouldn't smoke; it will kill you."

We both just sat in the chairs until the sun came up.

As we packed up our gear in relative silence, preparing for my last day on safari, Adnan reached into his pack and produced a walkie-talkie that I previously was not aware was in his possession. He had a quick exchange with someone on the other line in his native tongue; then he finished extinguishing the fire pit. About twenty minutes later and to my surprise, Adnan's driver showed up with the Jeep. Adnan started to throw the gear into the Jeep and motioned me to come over.

"Mr. Scott, I want to take you to my village today if you agree. It is the late-summer harvest celebration, and some of my family will be there." I quickly nodded in approval. Considering the previous few days of excitement, I thought it would be a very welcome and relaxing breather before my departure. After about a fifteen-minute trek through the bush, we came upon what appeared to be a heavily traversed main road and were able to travel much faster than I had been used to in the last three days. We spent about forty-five minutes on the Tanzanian version of a freeway, a dirt road, taking in the African landscape for one last time.

Once again we left the relative comfort of the well-traveled road and headed east on what looked to be another tractor path. After another ten-minute drive, we came upon what appeared to be a large farm full of crops, with cattle grazing in a neighboring field. As we neared the village, we passed both traditional thatched huts, common to the Sukuma people, and larger mortar-and-brick buildings made from the native clay and soil, capped with rusty metal roofs. As we approached a spacious clearing, and what seemed to be the center of the village, there were a large number of villagers lined up around the perimeter of the village square. Numbering in the hundreds, they were both seated next to and standing against the brick buildings, obviously waiting for some sort of event or spectacle. The Jeep came to a stop, and a handful of small children ran to greet us, wondering I'm sure who this new and strangely pale visitor might be…

Adnan exited the Jeep and welcomed the children with open arms, pointing toward me and giving them what seemed to be some instructions in their native tongue of Bantu. With Adnan motioning me over, I exited the Jeep, and the children grabbed both my hands and led me toward a bench under a tree between two of the thatched huts. Adnan eventually came over to sit next to me and remarked that we had gotten here just in time.

Just then I heard whistles blowing from behind the huts, and everyone stood, jumping and clapping in excitement. Adnan explained that this time of year was an ancient and highly celebrated time for their people, the late-summer harvest. The whistles now got louder, and then a group of Sukuma men near one of the brick buildings started pounding loudly on drums in rhythmic harmony. Out from behind the huts marched a parade of men and women villagers dressed in traditional robes, dancing to the beat of the large drums while blowing whistles and waving feathers weaved together on a stick. The women were chanting and playing what seemed to be finger symbols, and toward the end of the parade of villagers, a group of the Sukuma men carried two large boxes into the center of the gathering. Two distinct groups now separated dancing around the two individual boxes.

Adnan explained as the procession passed us that this was an important part of the ancient rituals dating back centuries. It started with two distinct neighboring tribes during the harvest season. Each tribe would visit the other, sending a group to represent their individual tribe that consisted of their most highly revered dancers and medicine men. The Sukuma are a very spiritual and superstitious people, believing in the power of magic and spirits. The legend that was passed down from generation to generation was that each dance group from those ancient tribes were lathered up with their medicine man's most potent and magical medicine...and the winner of the competition would be judged and determined by which tribe's dance group drew the largest crowd, having been drawn to them, as the legend goes, by which tribe had the most powerful and magical medicines. This tradition morphed over the generations, and while not losing the tradition of the medicine men, an element of showmanship was introduced in an attempt to win the largest crowds. This led to more and more outrageous acts, theatrics, and modes of dress as the years progressed…and I was about to witness how far this elevation of showmanship and outrageousness had progressed into modern times. As the two separate groups danced in circles vying for the attention of the crowd, the men who had carried in the large boxes quickly uncovered them simultaneously, while the whistle blowing grew louder, and the feather shaking intensified.

One man from each group then reached into the two boxes and pulled out by the tail the most enormous pythons I had ever seen, neither in a zoo nor on television. They easily exceeded fifteen feet in total length, along with attaining nearly the girth of a telephone pole.

Now, the tribesmen pulling them out of the boxes, I was soon to learn, was far from being the most outrageous part. I nudged Adnan in the ribs. "I haven't seen enough snakes for one trip?"

Just then one of the men, whom Adnan had pointed out as being his cousin, grabbed the python by the tail, wrapping him around his neck, still dancing the whole time. While the snake's menacing triangular head bobbed about, glancing off his feet and thighs, there was absolutely no consideration for whether or not the snake might sink his huge fangs deep into his flesh.

"I thought it was important you see this after last night," Adnan professed. "You will see my people have learned not to fear them." Just as he said this and perfectly exemplifying his point, Adnan's cousin grabbed that enormous snake by the head, forced the python's jaws shut, and stuffed as much of that snake's head as possible directly into his own mouth, dancing all the while. After about ten seconds he released the snake from his clutches and the snake slithered back into his box, almost on command.

"I wanted to show you, Mr. Scott, with all that you have to fear right now in your life…that you must not let your fear win; you must look fear straight in the eyes and say, 'I will eat you…you will not eat me.'" His wisdom hit me like a ton of bricks. I put my head down, fighting off more emotion than I had even experienced the night before, being seconds away from certain death.

We enjoyed the rest of the parade and dance competition. Afterward he introduced me to his family, along with a quick tour of the village. He showed me the crops his family grew, primarily maize, vegetables, and cotton, which they sold as a cash crop. It was now getting later in the day, and it came time for me to depart for my plane to Dar es Salaam. Adnan instructed his driver to go through my things and make sure all my bags were there. Once everything was accounted for, Adnan accompanied me to the Jeep and gave me a big hug. As we released from our embrace, he held on to both my shoulders and said something I still carry with me to this day.

"Mr. Scott, the Sukuma have a very famous and ancient proverb that I want you to remember and that we live by every day—*the wind cannot break a tree that bends.*" Adnan bowed his head, gathering his thoughts. He finally looked up and, while staring at me with an air of confidence, said, "Just remember, this may bend you…but it will never break you."

We embraced again. I thanked him for everything he had done for me and explained how impactful and inspirational he had been to me in just a few short days. We said our good-byes, and I was off to the airstrip…and once again on my way home and back to reality.

Chapter 5

CONCLUSION

Reach further than the grasp you are comfortable with…

How could I ever let my day-to-day anxieties affect me again? When I get that pit-of-my-stomach cringe just before I am about to board a plane, I remember that I braved the perils of one of the most challenging volcanic cliffs Hawaii has to offer. When I am once again lying on that MRI bed, and it starts eerily creeping forward into that confined space with all the violent buzzing, clicks, and alarms…I remind myself that I was face-to-face in a death stare with a black mamba. How dare you let this little minor inconvenience during the course of a day give you even a twinge of nervousness?

And then it disappears, as quickly as it came. The routine and primarily mundane anxieties I had experienced for decades suddenly vanish… not with Xanax, not with a psychologist and some herbal tea, and not with a jog or breathing into a brown paper bag. No, the choice that I made to live my life made all the debilitating worry and anxiety drain out of my body, like water out of a freshly wrung sponge. And like a dry sponge, it was eager to absorb something to fill its void. I filled that void with irreplaceable memories and adventure that can never evaporate like those anxieties did. And now these stories and adventures will live on for my family to remember and relive.

So take that first step.

Hit the gas instead of the brake.

Go up to that girl, and ask her to dance.

Go on that exotic vacation, and keep a journal.

You must make this life count for something.

Face your anxiety, and it will all quickly disappear.

A tree that bends cannot be broken.

Never let fear determine your fate…

Choose to live.